The Most Common Inpatient Problems in Internal Medicine

JOHN C. SUN, MD
San Francisco, California

HYLTON V. JOFFE, MD
Washington, District of Columbia

D1628450

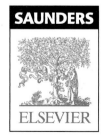

SAUNDERS

ELSEVIER

SAUNDERS
ELSEVIER

1600 John F. Kennedy Blvd, Suite 1800
Philadelphia, Pennsylvania 19103–2899

The Most Common Inpatient Problems in Internal Medicine
ISBN-13: 978-1-4160-3203-8
ISBN-10: 1-4160-3203-7

Notice

Knowledge and best practice in this field of Internal Medicine
are constantly changing. As new research and experience
broaden our knowledge, changes in practice, treatment and drug
therapy may become necessary or appropriate. Readers are
advised to check the most current information provided (i) on
procedures featured or (ii) by the manufacturer of each product
to be administered, to verify the recommended dose or formula,
the method and duration of administration, and contraindications. It is the responsibility of the practitioner, relying on their
own experience and knowledge of the patient, to make diagnoses,
to determine dosages and the best treatment for each individual
patient, and to take all appropriate safety precautions. To the
fullest extent of the law, neither the Publisher nor the Editors
assumes any liability for any injury and/or damage to persons or
property arising out of or related to any use of the material con-
tained in this book.

The Publisher

International Standard Book Number 1-4160-3203-7

Editor: Rolla Couchman
Developmental Editor: Adrianne Brigido
Design Direction: Gene Harris

Printed in the United States of America.

Last digit is the print number: 9 8 7 6 5 4 3 2 1

Acknowledgments

We learned a tremendous amount about inpatient medicine during our internship and residency. We are indebted to the many talented colleagues, residents, chief residents, fellows, and staff physicians with whom we worked during those formative years. We especially thank Dr. Joel Katz, the Program Director for the Internal Medicine training program at Brigham and Women's Hospital who constantly strives to improve the residency program and who has kindly agreed to write a foreword for this book. We also thank Dr. Marshall Wolf, a master clinician-educator, for believing in us and granting us the privilege of training at one of the best hospitals in the country. We thank Rolla Couchman and Dylan Parker, our contacts at Elsevier, for their expertise, guidance, professionalism, and patience as we worked toward meeting deadlines. Without them, this book would still be a figment of our imagination and not this work of which we are both very proud.

John Sun would like to thank Dr. David Katzka and Dr. Anil Rustgi for their outstanding teaching and mentorship. He also thanks his parents, his brother, Alan, and his extended family for their encouragement. Most importantly, he thanks his wife, Yumee, for her many years of dedication, love, and support.

Hylton Joffe would like to thank Dr. Samuel Goldhaber, Dr. Arthur Sasahara, and Dr. Robert Utiger—phenomenal role models as physicians, mentors, and human beings. He also thanks his parents, his sister, Karen, and his brother-in-law, Daniel, for their encouragement and love. Most of all, he thanks his wife, Sarah, for her unselfish, unwavering, and unconditional love and support.

Foreword

According to the eminent medical educator, Dr. Marshall Wolf, the fundamental skill required to master the Art of Medicine is the ability to accurately make critical—often life-sustaining—decisions in the face of incomplete data. Every trainee and practicing physician will encounter common medical conditions with a high degree of regularity, and needs an approach to clinical decision-making that is reflexive and yet retains the nuanced recognition of the subtleties affecting the individual patient. Skilled providers must have, at the same time, a command of practical, evidence-based management strategies as well as an appreciation of the guideposts requiring individual variations. The latter skill comes only from experience. The former is the goal of this clear and authoritative volume.

Medical textbooks and handbooks play a vital role in the education of students, residents, fellows, and practicing physicians. This new contribution, *The Most Common Inpatient Problems in Internal Medicine,* is the result of collaboration between two truly gifted clinicians and teachers, Drs. John Sun and Hylton Joffe. Without abandoning subtlety, they have captured the key aspects of modern therapeutics in chapters addressing the most frequent and, therefore, most important acute medical problems. The text is organized for clarity, simplicity, and accessibility—critical commodities to the busy, and often over-stretched, physician-in-training. I predict with confidence that this volume will play a vital role in teaching and learning medicine. Future generations of students and teachers, and ultimately the patients they serve, will benefit from this important contribution.

Joel T. Katz, MD

Director
Internal Medicine Residency Program
Brigham and Women's Hospital
Member, Academy of Teaching Scholars
Assistant Professor of Medicine
Harvard Medical School
Boston, Massachusetts

Preface

Are you a medical student, intern, or resident who is (or will be) caring for patients on the medical ward? Do you find it challenging to locate practical and pertinent information about many of the common inpatient medical conditions? If your answers to these questions are "yes," then this book is for you!

Not too long ago, we were trying to learn the basic principles for the day-to-day care of medical inpatients. We found that review articles and book chapters provided an overview of medical topics but often lacked specific information directly applicable to patient care. Frequently, we also had difficulty determining the relevance of findings from original journal articles, especially when there were prior conflicting studies. As a result, we learned a vast amount of practical inpatient medicine from our co-interns, residents, fellows, and staff physicians. These teachers explained how to choose a dose of intravenous furosemide for our patient with decompensated heart failure or how to calculate the dose of subcutaneous insulin for a patient with resolving diabetic ketoacidosis. Basic concepts such as these have often been frustratingly difficult to acquire from other sources. Until now.

Our book, *The Most Common Inpatient Problems in Internal Medicine,* provides practical and pertinent information for the most common medical problems encountered on the hospital ward. The chapters cover basic principles that every house officer should know, emphasizing "bread-and-butter" medicine. You will find useful information about common disorders you see everyday, including heart failure, pancreatitis, hyperkalemia, acute exacerbation of chronic obstructive pulmonary disease, asthma, acute renal failure, hyponatremia, and unstable angina. After reading this book, you will have a solid foundation upon which to build your knowledge as you advance in your career.

You will find answers to the following types of questions:

- What rate and type of intravenous fluid should I administer to my patient with acute, symptomatic hyponatremia?
- Does my patient have iron deficiency anemia or anemia of chronic disease?
- How do I teach my patient with chronic obstructive pulmonary disease to use a spacer for delivery of her inhaled glucocorticoids?
- How do I differentiate aspiration pneumonia from chemical pneumonitis and do these patients require antibiotics?
- How can I determine whether my patient's renal failure is acute or chronic when prior serum creatinine measurements are unavailable?
- My patient with suspected pulmonary embolism has a normal first-generation lung computed tomography (CT) scan—what should I do next?

Each chapter is divided into sections that cover the epidemiology, pathophysiology, signs and symptoms, laboratory abnormalities, diagnosis, and management of the disorder under discussion. A "Key Points" box at the beginning of each chapter highlights some important take-home messages. Tables and figures clarify important and complex concepts. Each chapter ends with a list of references, which can also be used by those who wish to further their knowledge in specific areas.

We hope that you will enjoy reading this book as much as we enjoyed writing it.

Best of luck in your career!

John C. Sun, MD
San Francisco, California

Hylton V. Joffe, MD
Washington, District of Columbia

About the Authors

Dr. John C. Sun received his medical education at Temple University where he was elected to the Alpha Omega Alpha Honor Society during his junior year. Dr. Sun received the Golden Stethoscope Award for outstanding teaching during his internal medicine training at Brigham and Women's Hospital and Harvard Medical School. After residency, Dr. Sun completed a Gastroenterology fellowship at the University of Pennsylvania, where he served on the Gastroenterology Education Committee. He is currently a gastroenterologist at Kaiser Permanente, San Francisco, and participates in medical student teaching at the University of California, San Francisco. He lives in San Francisco with his wife, Yumee, and son, Ethan.

Dr. Hylton V. Joffe received his medical education at the University of Arizona where he was elected to the Alpha Omega Alpha Honor Society during his junior year. Dr. Joffe received recognition from the internship class for excellence in teaching during his internal medicine training at Brigham and Women's Hospital and Harvard Medical School. After residency, Dr. Joffe completed an Endocrinology fellowship at Brigham and Women's Hospital and received formal training in Clinical Investigation through the Scholars in Clinical Science Program at Harvard Medical School. He is currently a Medical Officer in the Division of Metabolism and Endocrinology Products at the U.S. Food and Drug Administration as well as a member of the Division of Endocrinology and Metabolism at the Johns Hopkins University School of Medicine. Dr. Joffe lives in Washington, DC, with his wife, Sarah.

Table of Contents

SECTION V INFECTIOUS DISEASES

SECTION VI PULMONARY

SECTION VII RENAL

SECTION I

Cardiology

CHAPTER 1

Atrial Fibrillation

KEY POINTS

1. Atrial fibrillation is an irregular supraventricular arrhythmia that may cause thromboembolism, hypotension, and cardiac ischemia or infarction.
2. Risk factors for thromboembolism include increasing age, prior history of thromboembolic events, hypertension, heart failure, and diabetes mellitus.
3. Evaluation of a patient with atrial fibrillation includes a history and physical examination to assess the timing and duration of symptoms, potential triggers or reversible causes, and presence of complications.
4. Basic laboratory testing, thyroid function tests, electrocardiogram, echocardiography, and chest x-ray should be performed.
5. Rate-control or rhythm-control strategies have similar thromboembolism rates. Both require anticoagulation to decrease the risk of embolic events.
6. Most patients should be treated using rate-control. Rhythm control should be reserved for patients who prefer rhythm-control, have continued symptoms despite adequate rate control, or fail to achieve rate control.
7. Acute rate control may be achieved with intravenous metoprolol, verapamil, or diltiazem (see text for dosing). Digoxin should not be used.
8. Beta-blockers, calcium channel blockers (verapamil, diltiazem), or digoxin may be used for chronic rate control.

> Beta-blockers and calcium channel
> blockers will provide rate control at rest
> and with exercise. Digoxin provides rate
> control at rest, but not with exercise.

DEFINITION

Atrial fibrillation (Afib) is an irregularly
irregular supraventricular tachyarrhythmia
that results in loss of coordinated atrial
systole. The American College of Cardiology/
American Heart Association/European Society
of Cardiology (ACC/AHA/ESC) Practice
Guidelines define the following categories for
atrial fibrillation that lasts for longer than
30 seconds, and is not due to a reversible cause:

- Recurrent: Two or more episodes of Afib

- Paroxysmal: Recurrent Afib that termi-
  nates spontaneously (usually within 7 days)

- Persistent: Afib that is sustained (does not
  spontaneously resolve) for longer than 7
  days

- Permanent: Afib that lasts longer than
  1 year

- Lone Afib: Occurs in a patient:
  - Younger than 60 years of age
  - Without evidence of cardiac or pulmonary
    disease

EPIDEMIOLOGY

The prevalence of Afib increases with age, from
<1% in patients under age 60, to >6% in patients
above age 80. Afib is also more common in males
than in females, and in Caucasians than in African
Americans. The incidence for Afib is under
0.1% annually for persons under age 40, rising to

1.5% to 2% annually in persons over age 80. In a large study of almost 2 million members of a health maintenance organization (HMO), the overall prevalence of Afib was 1%, but ranged from 0.1% in patients under age 55 to 9% in patients over age 80. The prevalence of Afib also increases with the severity of heart failure.

The ischemic stroke risk for persons with nonvalvular Afib ranges from 2 to 7 times that of persons without Afib. For persons with rheumatic heart disease and Afib, the stroke risk is even higher, up to 17 times that of persons without Afib. For untreated patients, the stroke risk increases with age, from 1.5% annually in patients between the ages of 50 and 59, to 23.5% in patients between the ages of 80 and 89.

PATHOGENESIS

Potential Mechanisms

Afib is thought to be due to either enhanced automaticity of atrial foci or the presence of reentry circuits.

- Foci of enhanced automaticity:
  - Are usually located in the superior pulmonary veins.
  - May also be located in the right atrium, superior vena cava, or coronary sinus.
  - May be an important pathophysiologic mechanism in paroxysmal Afib.
- Reentry circuits:
  - May be numerous, giving rise to differing numbers of wavelets of depolarization.
  - Are related to atrial size, refractory period, and conduction velocities.

The success rate of cardioversion for Afib is the highest within the first 24 hours of onset of Afib. With longer duration of Afib, electrophysiological remodeling occurs, resulting in decreased atrial refractory periods and perhaps increasing the sinus node recovery time. In addition, prolonged duration of Afib may result in an increased recovery time for atrial contractility after cardioversion.

Afib is often initiated by other supraventricular arrhythmias or atrial premature beats. Atrioventricular (AV) nodal reentry and atrioventricular reentry tachycardias may also result in Afib.

Pathophysiologic Effects

Ventricular Rate

Conduction of electrical impulses to the ventricle via the AV node is related to autonomic tone, AV nodal refractory period, and concealed conduction (atrial impulses may enter the AV node, but are not transmitted to the ventricle).

- There is an inverse relationship between the atrial and ventricular rates. Higher atrial rates are associated with lower ventricular rates, and lower atrial rates are associated with higher ventricular rates.
- Increased parasympathetic and decreased sympathetic tone decrease conduction across the AV node. Decreased parasympathetic tone and increased sympathetic tone increase conduction across the AV node.

Hemodynamic Effects

Afib results in the loss of atrial systole (causing decreased ventricular filling) and the potential for a rapid ventricular response. Both have the potential to lower cardiac output.

Loss of atrial systole may have pronounced consequences in patients with decreased ventricular compliance (i.e., left ventricular hypertrophy, hypertrophic cardiomyopathy) or mitral stenosis.

Rapid ventricular response to Afib may result in decreased cardiac output due to lack of ventricular filling time compounded by loss of atrioventricular synchrony and suboptimal contractility.

Over time, atrial and ventricular tachycardia result in atrial and dilated ventricular cardiomyopathy, respectively. Atrial cardiomyopathy leads to decreased myocyte contractility and propensity for the development of sustained Afib. Ventricular cardiomyopathy may lead to signs and symptoms of heart failure. Both are potentially reversible with control of Afib.

Embolic Complications

Thrombus formation tends to occur in the left atrial appendage, accessible to examination by transesophageal echocardiography. Although the precise mechanism of thrombus formation remains unclear, a combination of decreased blood flow through the atrial appendage and regional coagulopathy likely play a role.

Risk factors for stroke in patients with Afib include:

- Hypertension: Patients with hypertension and Afib have lower flow rates through the left atrial appendage and higher associated thrombus formation.
- Increasing age: Older patients with Afib tend to have left atrial enlargement and lower left atrial appendage flow rates, resulting in a higher risk of thrombus formation.
- Left ventricular systolic dysfunction: Heart failure is associated with a higher stroke risk in patients with Afib.

Risk Factors and Potential Causes

Patients without Cardiac Disease

Metabolic factors (such as obesity and hyperthyroidism) and drugs (such as adenosine, theophylline, and alcohol) may cause Afib. Noncardiac (particularly thoracic) surgery may induce Afib. Pulmonary embolism, chronic obstructive pulmonary disease, and obstructive sleep apnea are associated with Afib, as well. Obstructive sleep apnea does not initiate Afib but has been found to increase the risk of Afib recurrence.

Autonomic dysfunction may be associated with Afib. Vagally mediated Afib tends to occur during periods of heightened parasympathetic tone, such as mealtimes, or during sleep. Adrenergically mediated Afib usually happens during the day, with exercise, or during emotional or physical stress.

Patients with Cardiac Disease

Hypertension, coronary artery disease, and valvular heart disease are the most common cardiac disorders associated with Afib, and are found in roughly 21%, 17%, and 15% of patients with Afib, respectively. Afib is an unusual presentation of cardiac ischemia or infarction, with the latter occurring in 5.5% of patients seen in an emergency department. For valvular heart disease, mitral valve disorders have a higher association with Afib than do aortic valve disorders.

Other cardiac diseases associated with Afib include hypertrophic cardiomyopathy, heart failure, pericarditis, myocarditis, presence of other supraventricular arrhythmias, cor pulmonale, cardiac surgery, and transplantation.

CLINICAL FEATURES AND EVALUATION

Patients most commonly complain of palpitations, lightheadedness, fatigue, chest pain, or dyspnea. However, many episodes of Afib are asymptomatic. The physical examination may reveal an irregularly irregular pulse, varying intensity of the first heart sound, or murmurs associated with valvular disease.

The ACC/AHA/ESC Practice Guidelines present a coherent plan for the evaluation of the patient with Afib, described in the following text:

History and Physical Examination

The history should attempt to determine:

- Time of initial diagnosis or onset of symptoms of Afib
- Frequency, duration, and potential precipitating causes of Afib
- Method of termination of Afib, including spontaneous resolution or pharmacologic therapy
- Presence of other symptoms due to Afib

Particular attention should be placed on determining if any of the risk factors or potential causes described in the prior section apply to the patient.

- Alcohol and medication use should be determined. Precipitation of Afib with alcohol intake may also suggest vagal-mediated Afib, particularly if it also occurs at night or during meals.
- Findings of heat intolerance, modest weight loss, changes in hair or skin texture, or hyperreflexia should suggest hyperthyroidism. However, many patients may have subclinical thyroid disease.
- Dyspnea, history of tobacco use, hyperinflation, wheezing, or decreased breath sounds may be consistent with chronic obstructive pulmonary disease. Pleuritic chest pain, dyspnea with lower extremity swelling, and a recent history of prolonged immobilization suggest a pulmonary embolus.
- Evidence of cardiac disease, including hypertension, heart failure, history of supraventricular arrhythmias, or valvular disease should be sought.

Laboratory and Other Tests

A 12-lead electrocardiogram (EKG) should be obtained to ascertain the diagnosis of Afib. An EKG may also reveal evidence of cardiac ischemia, prior myocardial infarction, presence of other arrhythmias, and left ventricular hypertrophy.

A chest x-ray should be obtained to evaluate the pulmonary parenchyma, vasculature, and cardiac silhouette.

Transthoracic echocardiography (TTE) should be performed. TTE can assess atrial size, ventricular size and function, and evaluate for valvular heart disease, pulmonary hypertension, and pericardial disease. Although TTE may show left atrial thrombus formation, it is not the diagnostic test of choice. A transesophageal echocardiogram (TEE) should be performed to definitively assess for the presence of left atrial thrombi.

Thyroid function tests should be obtained to assess for hyperthyroidism.

Further Testing

Holter Monitor and Exercise Tests

Holter monitoring may be helpful to establish the diagnosis in patients with signs and symptoms consistent with Afib, but in whom a routine EKG is unrevealing (i.e., paroxysmal Afib). Exercise testing may reveal associated cardiac ischemia in patients with Afib. In addition, both Holter monitoring and exercise testing may be used to determine whether a patient's rate control is sufficient.

Transesophageal Echocardiography (TEE)

The major role of TEE is to assess for left atrial or left atrial appendage thrombus. This may be useful to determine whether there is an atrial thrombus in patients with ischemic stroke, or prior to cardioversion. In patients with Afib for longer than 48 hours, use of TEE to exclude an atrial thrombus prior to cardioversion resulted in similar thromboembolism rates ($<1\%$) compared with traditional anticoagulation strategies, which use 3 to 4 weeks of anticoagulation prior to cardioversion.

Electrophysiological Study (EP Study)

EP studies may be utilized in patients who are candidates for catheter ablation, AV conduction modification, or pacemaker placement as potential treatments for Afib.

TREATMENT

Overview

The major issues in the management of Afib are:

- Should a rate-control or rhythm-control strategy be used?
- What is the best method to decrease the risk of thromboembolism?
- How should patients with recent onset of Afib be managed?
- Which patients should be considered for urgent cardioversion?

Rate or Rhythm Control?

Theoretically, maintenance of normal sinus rhythm should be the optimal strategy, should decrease the risk of thromboembolism, and should result in better overall outcomes. However, two major studies, the Atrial Fibrillation Follow-Up Investigation of Rhythm Management (AFFIRM) and Rate Control versus Electrical Cardioversion for Persistent Atrial Fibrillation (RACE) trials, demonstrated that there is no significant difference in the embolic risk between a rate-control and a rhythm-control strategy. This is likely due to:

- Recurrence of Afib in patients after cardioversion, with most episodes being asymptomatic.
- Presence of other risk factors for thromboembolism, such as atherosclerosis or heart failure.

Therefore, anticoagulation should be used regardless of whether a rate-control or rhythm-control strategy is chosen.

In addition, there was a trend to increased mortality for the rhythm-control arm of the AFFIRM trial, which is likely due to medication-related adverse events. The RACE trial also showed a trend toward higher nonfatal adverse outcomes in the rhythm-control arm.

The results of these studies suggest that there is no significant benefit to a rhythm-control strategy in terms of need for anticoagulation or overall outcomes. Thus, the American Academy of Family Physicians/American College of Physicians (AAFP/ACP) guidelines (2003) recommend that a rate-control strategy with anticoagulation be used for most patients. A rhythm control strategy should be reserved for:

- Patients who continue to have angina, heart failure, dyspnea, or other symptoms despite achieving good rate control (see following text for parameters of adequate rate control)
- Patients who fail to achieve good rate control
- Patients who prefer a rhythm-control strategy

A limitation of the already cited studies is that the average patient age was over 68 years old. These results may not be generalizable to young, otherwise healthy patients. As a result, some experts may attempt cardioversion in younger patients with a reversible cause of Afib (such as pericarditis, hyperthyroidism, or pulmonary embolism), and without hypertension, heart disease, or left atrial enlargement (left atrial size should be <4.5 cm).

Rate Control

As has been mentioned, there is no statistically significant difference in overall mortality or rate of embolic events between a rate-control and rhythm-control strategy. Both methods require anticoagulation to decrease the risk of thromboembolism. We will describe pharmacologic methods for rate control here. A discussion of nonpharmacologic approaches to rate control is beyond the scope of this chapter.

Targets for rate control differ among different patient populations. For example, a sedentary patient with heart failure may require only control of ventricular rate at rest, whereas an active, younger patient may require adequate control of ventricular rate during exercise. The AFFIRM trial used the following criteria to define successful rate control:

- Resting average heart rate <80 bpm
- Either one of the following:
  - Maximum heart rate during a 6-minute walk <100 bpm, or
  - Average heart rate <100 bpm during 24-hour Holter monitor, *and* heart rate <110% of maximum predicted heart rate for patient's age at all times

The ACC/AHA/ESC guidelines state that ventricular rate should be maintained between 60 and 80 bpm at rest, and between 90 and 115 bpm with moderate exercise. Practically speaking, the goal is to achieve symptom control during a patient's routine daily activities.

Medications used to achieve rate control fall into three groups:

- Beta-blocking agents, such as metoprolol or atenolol
  - Control ventricular rate at rest and during exercise
  - Beneficial in patients with Afib and heart failure, myocardial ischemia, or infarction
  - Should be used with caution in patients with pulmonary disease such as asthma
- Calcium channel blockers, such as verapamil and diltiazem

- Control ventricular rate at rest and during exercise
- Use with caution in patients with heart failure or second- or third-degree AV block
- Verapamil increases the serum digoxin level
- Digoxin:
  - Controls ventricular rate at rest. Lacks efficacy for control of ventricular rate during exercise
  - Should not be used as first-line therapy for rate control except in patients with Afib and heart failure
  - Has a slow onset of action and should not be used for acute rate control

Overall, the most effective regimen appears to be combination therapy with beta-blockers and digoxin. For monotherapy, beta-blockers are more effective than calcium channel blockers, and digoxin is the least effective. None of the three medications should be used in patients with Wolff-Parkinson-White syndrome.

Acute Therapy

Both beta-blockers and calcium channel blockers may be used for acute therapy of rapid ventricular rate. Digoxin should not be used, because it has an onset of action up to 60 minutes from time of infusion.

- Metoprolol:
  - Give 2.5–5 mg IV over 2 min
  - May repeat every 5 min, as needed
  - Maximum IV dose is 15 mg
- Verapamil:
  - Give 5–10 mg IV over 2 min
  - May repeat every 15 min, as needed
  - Once rate control is achieved, may give continuous infusion of 0.125 mg/min to maintain rate control
- Diltiazem:

- For initial dose, give 0.25 mg/kg body weight IV over 2 min.
- After 15 min, repeat with 0.35 mg/kg body weight given over 2 min, if necessary.
- In patients who respond to either 1 or 2 IV bolus doses, start maintenance infusion of 5 to 15 mg IV per hour.

Chronic Therapy

Long-term ventricular rate control may be achieved with oral doses of beta-blockers, calcium channel blockers, digoxin, or a combination of the previously mentioned drugs:

- Metoprolol: 25–100 mg orally twice a day
- Atenolol: 25–100 mg orally daily
- Verapamil: 40–120 mg orally three times a day
- Diltiazem: 30–90 mg orally four times a day
- Digoxin: 0.25 mg orally every 2 hr up to 1.5 mg total loading dose, then 0.125–0.375 mg orally daily. Digoxin levels should be monitored at about 1 week when steady levels are achieved, or when digoxin toxicity is suspected.

In patients with rapid ventricular rate despite treatment with these medications, amiodarone may be used for rate control:

- Amiodarone: 800 mg orally daily for 1 week, followed by 600 mg daily for 1 week, then 400 mg daily for 4–6 weeks.
- Amiodarone: 200 mg orally daily as maintenance may then be continued after the loading regimen is completed.

Due to the significant side effects, amiodarone should be initiated after consultation with a cardiologist.

Rhythm Control

Results from the AFFIRM and RACE trials show no significant difference in rates of embolic events between rate and rhythm control strategies. There may be a trend toward decreased overall mortality in patients treated with rate-control. Therefore, rhythm control is reserved for patients who:

- Fail an adequate trial of rate control:
  - Patients who have continued symptoms despite good rate control.
  - Patients who continue to have rapid ventricular response despite use of maximal pharmacologic rate control.
  - Patients who fail rate control may need to be maintained on anti-arrhythmic medications.
  - Patients who fail rate may also be considered for nonpharmacologic treatment of Afib, including catheter ablation.
- Prefer a rhythm control strategy
  - Routine use of anti-arrhythmic medications not recommended by the AAFP/ACP guidelines
  - Anticoagulation is recommended.
  - If rhythm control is unsuccessful in these patients, rate-control is recommended.
- Have an initial episode of Afib
  - Routine use of anti-arrhythmic medications not recommended by the AAFP/ACP guidelines
  - Anticoagulation is recommended.
  - If rhythm control is unsuccessful, initiation of rate-control is recommended
- Have Afib associated with symptoms and signs of hypotension, heart failure, myocardial ischemia, or infarction despite maximal rate control
  - In the acute setting, these patients should be considered for emergent cardioversion.

Methods of Cardioversion

Either electrical or pharmacologic cardioversion may be used. Electrical cardioversion is accomplished using a synchronized direct current delivered via electrodes on the patient's thorax. Pharmacologic cardioversion is achieved using antiarrhythmic medications. Both methods require appropriate anticoagulation or TEE, discussed in the section on prevention of thromboembolism. Although a detailed analysis of cardioversion is beyond the scope of this chapter (the reader is referred to the ACC/AHA/ESC guidelines listed in the following text), a brief discussion follows. Cardioversion should be performed by an experienced cardiologist.

Electrical Cardioversion

Electrical cardioversion is more effective than pharmacologic cardioversion, and is usually the method of choice. The patient is asked to fast overnight and is given conscious sedation prior to the procedure. Subsequently, electrode pads or paddles are placed either in the anterior–posterior (sternum anteriorly and left subscapular position posteriorly) or anterior–lateral (right subclavicular anteriorly and ventricular apex laterally) positions. Some data suggest that the anterior–posterior configuration may result in a higher success rate compared to the anterior–lateral configuration.

For monophasic waveform, an initial energy setting of 200 J, synchronized with the QRS complex should be used. The energy may be increased by 100 J for additional shocks, to a maximum of 400 J. A minimum of 1 minute should elapse between successive shocks to minimize myocardial damage. The success rate for electrical cardioversion is between 70% and 90%.

The major risks associated with electrical cardioversion are thromboembolism, myocardial damage, and arrhythmias. Embolic events occur in 1% to 7% of patients; this risk may be decreased with appropriate anticoagulation prior to cardioversion. The risk of myocardial damage is usually not clinically significant. Benign arrhythmias, including premature beats, bradycardia, and short sinus pauses may commonly occur after cardioversion. Patients with abnormal potassium or digitalis levels are at risk for the development of ventricular tachycardia or fibrillation; potassium and digoxin levels should be determined prior to cardioversion. Sinus node dysfunction may be present in patients with chronic Afib. These patients often have normal ventricular rates without the use of pharmacologic rate control. Prophylactic pacemaker use may be considered in these patients prior to cardioversion.

Pharmacologic Cardioversion

Pharmacologic cardioversion is more effective if used within 7 days of onset of Afib, and therefore is often used for an initial episode of Afib. It is less effective for patients with persistent Afib and those with Afib of longer than 7 days' duration.

The major side effects of pharmacologic cardioversion are thromboembolism and arrhythmias. Up to 13% of patients may experience arrhythmias, with bradycardia being the most common. Other cardiac-related adverse events include heart failure, hypotension, and conduction abnormalities. The risk is higher in patients with prior myocardial infarction.

The ACC/AHA/ESC guidelines state that dofetilide, flecainide, propafenone, ibutilide, and amiodarone are efficacious in patients with Afib of less than 7 days' duration, while dofetilide, ibutilide and amiodarone may be useful in patients with Afib of longer than 7 days' duration.

Prevention of Thromboembolism

As has been stated, the stroke risk for patients with Afib is two to seven times that of age-adjusted controls and is higher in older patients. Use of aspirin or warfarin with a target International Normalized Ratio (INR) of at least 2.0 to 3.0 lowers the risk of thromboembolic events in patients with Afib. Risk factors for thromboembolism include a history of thromboembolism, hypertension, increasing age, diabetes mellitus, coronary artery disease, hyperthyroidism, and female sex.

Chronic Prevention

Patients should be risk-stratified to determine appropriate therapy to prevent thromboembolism. The ACC/AHA/ESC guidelines recommend:

- Aspirin 325 mg orally daily for
  - patients under age 60 with heart disease but without risk factors of heart failure, hypertension, or left ventricular ejection fraction less than 35%
  - Patients older than 60 without risk factors
  - Patients under age 60 without heart disease or risk factors for thromboembolism may be treated with aspirin 325 mg orally daily, or no therapy
- Warfarin therapy should be offered, in the absence of contraindications, for patients who do not fall into these categories. Specifically,
  - Target INR 2.0–3.0 for patients with:
    - Age >60 with diabetes mellitus or coronary artery disease; Additional low-dose aspirin therapy optional
    - Age >75, particularly females
    - Heart failure with left ventricular ejection fraction less than 35%
    - Hypertension or thyrotoxicosis
  - Target INR 2.5–3.5 for patients with:
    - Rheumatic heart disease or mitral stenosis
    - Prosthetic heart valves
    - Prior thromboembolism
    - Persistent atrial thrombus on TEE

The CHADS2 scoring system is another risk stratification method. The CHADS2 values are assigned as follows:

- Congestive heart failure—1 point
- Hypertension—1 point
- Age >75—1 point

- Diabetes mellitus—1 point
- Secondary prevention for prior history of thromboembolism—2 points

Therapy should be administered as follows:

- CHADS2 score of 0—low risk of thromboembolism. Aspirin therapy may be used if no contraindications exist.
- CHADS2 score >3—high risk of thromboembolism. Warfarin therapy should be used if no contraindications exist.
- CHADS2 score of 2 in a patient with prior history of thromboembolism—high risk of thromboembolism. Warfarin therapy should be used if no contraindications exist.
- CHADS2 score of 1 to 2—intermediate risk of thromboembolism. Determination of aspirin or warfarin therapy should be guided by other clinical factors and patient preference.

Anticoagulation and Cardioversion

Patients with Afib of less than 48 hours' duration and no risk factors for thromboembolism (see preceding text) do not need 3 to 4 weeks of anticoagulation prior to cardioversion. However, these patients should receive heparin (unfractionated or low molecular weight) before and during cardioversion, and anticoagulation (usually with warfarin) for at least 4 weeks after cardioversion.

Afib of less than 48 hours' duration in a patient with significant risk factors for thromboembolism, including prior thromboembolic event, valvular heart disease, or heart failure, should receive 3 to 4 weeks of warfarin therapy prior to cardioversion. These patients should be maintained on warfarin for at least 4 weeks after cardioversion.

Afib of unknown or greater than 48 hours' duration may be managed with either:

- Prolonged anticoagulation:

- Patient is given 3–4 weeks of warfarin therapy, with a target INR of 2.5 (goal 2.0–3.0) prior to cardioversion.
- Lower risk of thromboembolic events is seen with an INR > 2.5 on the day of cardioversion.
- Anticoagulation should be maintained for at least 4 weeks after cardioversion.
- TEE-based strategy:
  - Heparin should be started and/or warfarin initiated for anticoagulation.
  - Transesophageal echocardiogram should then be performed. If a clot is visualized, or if a clot cannot be excluded, 3 to 4 weeks of anticoagulation should be given prior to cardioversion (as has been described). If a clot is excluded, cardioversion may be performed.
  - Anticoagulation should be maintained for a minimum of 4 weeks after cardioversion.

REFERENCES

Guidelines

1. Fuster V, Ryden LE, Asinger RW, et al. ACC/AHA/ESC guidelines for the management of patients with atrial fibrillation. *J Am Coll Cardiol.* 2001;38:1231–1266.
2. Snow V, Weiss KB, LeFevre M, et al. Management of newly detected atrial fibrillation: A clinical practice guideline from the American Academy of Family Physicians and the American College of Physicians. *Ann Int Med.* 2003;139:1009–1017.
3. Singer DE, Albers GW, Dalen JE, et al. Antithrombotic therapy in atrial fibrillation: The Seventh ACCP Conference on Antithrombotic and Thrombolytic Therapy. *Chest* 2004;126:429S–456S.

Review Articles

1. Page RL. Clinical practice. Newly diagnosed atrial fibrillation. *N Engl J Med*. 2004;351:2408–2416.
2. Falk RH. Atrial fibrillation. *N Engl J Med*. 2001;344:1067–1078.

Rate Control versus Rhythm Control

1. Van Gelder IC, Hagens VE, Bosker HA, et al. A comparison of rate control and rhythm control in patients with recurrent persistent atrial fibrillation. *N Engl J Med*. 2002;347:1834–1840.
2. Wyse DG, Waldo AL, DiMarco JP. A comparison of rate control and rhythm control in patients with atrial fibrillation. *N Engl J Med*. 2002;347:1825–1833.

Cardioversion and Anticoagulation

1. Gage BF, Waterman AD, Shannon W, et al. Validation of clinical classification schemes for predicting stroke: Results from the National Registry of Atrial Fibrillation. *JAMA* 2001;285:2864–2870.
2. Go AS, Hylek EM, Chang Y, et al. Anticoagulation therapy for stroke prevention in atrial fibrillation: How well do randomized trials translate into clinical practice? *JAMA* 2003;290:2685–2692.
3. Klein AL, Grimm RA, Murray RD, et al. Use of transesophageal echocardiography to guide cardioversion in patients with atrial fibrillation. *N Engl J Med*. 2001;344:1411–1420.
4. Weigner MJ, Caulfield TA, Danias PG, et al. Risk for clinical thromboembolism associated with conversion to sinus rhythm in patients with atrial fibrillation lasting less than 48 hours. *Ann Int Med*. 1997;126:615–620.

CHAPTER 2

Heart Failure

KEY POINTS

1. Systolic heart failure (HF) is caused by impaired ventricular ejection of blood. Diastolic HF results from impaired relaxation and filling of the left ventricle during diastole.
2. Symptomatic HF has a 1-year mortality of almost 50%.
3. The most common cause of HF is left ventricular systolic dysfunction, which typically results from coronary artery disease.
4. Symptoms of HF include dyspnea, orthopnea, paroxysmal nocturnal dyspnea, fatigue, exercise intolerance, peripheral edema, and weight gain.
5. Signs of HF include jugular venous distension, extra heart sounds (S_3 in left-sided HF and S_4 in patients with increased resistance to ventricular filling), pulmonary crackles, wheezing, pleural effusion, and pitting edema.
6. Initial testing should include electrolytes with blood urea nitrogen and creatinine, complete blood count, PA and lateral chest x-ray, electrocardiogram, and echocardiography. Cardiac catheterization is usually performed when no obvious cause for the HF is found or when myocardial ischemia is suspected.
7. Chest x-ray findings of HF may be obscured or distorted if there is underlying lung disease, and findings may be absent in patients with chronic HF.

8. HF is an unlikely cause of dyspnea in the emergency room when an untreated patient has normal levels of B-type natriuretic peptide.

9. Angiotensin-converting enzyme (ACE) inhibitors improve mortality, symptoms, left ventricular ejection fraction, and exercise tolerance and reduce hospitalizations. ACE inhibitors should be initiated early during the treatment of HF before excessive diuresis has occurred.

10. Patients who develop a cough or angioedema with ACE inhibitor therapy should be switched to an angiotensin receptor blocker (ARB).

11. Patients who develop significant renal insufficiency or hyperkalemia with ACE inhibitor or ARB therapy should be switched to combination hydralazine and isosorbide dinitrate.

12. Some beta-blockers such as carvedilol and bisoprolol improve morbidity and mortality in patients with HF, but should be initiated only after the patient's condition has stabilized and the volume status has been normalized.

13. Digoxin reduces hospitalization rates and improves symptoms and quality of life but does not lower mortality in patients with HF.

14. Mineralocorticoid receptor antagonists have shown promise in HF when used with ACE inhibitors but their concomitant use may be limited by hyperkalemia.

15. Clinical trials testing medications for diastolic HF are limited. ACE inhibitors and ARBs may improve exercise capacity and reduce the risk of hospitalization. Diuretics are appropriate for volume management but should be used

with caution because these patients are sensitive to excessive preload reduction.

16. Upon discharge, patients should be educated about dietary salt and fluid restriction and should weigh themselves daily on the same scale. Early identification and treatment of HF can reduce the likelihood of hospitalization.

DEFINITIONS

Heart failure (HF): Clinical syndrome characterized by signs and symptoms of volume overload and reduced organ perfusion.

Systolic heart failure: HF caused by impaired ventricular ejection of blood.

Diastolic heart failure: HF resulting from impaired relaxation and filling of the left ventricle during diastole. Diastolic HF can occur in patients with normal systolic function or can coexist with systolic HF. Since the normal lower limit of the ejection fraction is arbitrary, distinguishing between diastolic HF and systolic HF is sometimes difficult. At many medical facilities, an ejection fraction below 50% is considered abnormal.

EPIDEMIOLOGY

HF affects nearly 5 million Americans and accounts for at least 20% of hospital admissions among people over 65 years of age. Symptomatic HF has a 1-year mortality of almost 50%, conferring a worse prognosis than most cancers. As many as one-half of the patients with HF have normal or only minimally reduced systolic function, and are diagnosed with diastolic HF.

PATHOPHYSIOLOGY

Systolic Heart Failure

When the myocardium is weakened, the body attempts to maintain perfusion to vital organs by improving cardiac output and using systemic vasoconstriction to redistribute blood flow. Reduced renal perfusion leads to activation of the renin–angiotensin–aldosterone system, which causes extracellular volume expansion that raises end-diastolic volume and improves stroke volume via the Frank-Starling mechanism (this law states that increases in end-diastolic volume lead to increases in contractility and stroke volume). Catecholamines improve cardiac output by increasing heart rate and contractility. These compensatory neurohormonal mechanisms are initially beneficial but become deleterious over time. The systemic vasoconstriction increases the workload of the heart, which can lead to further myocardial deterioration. The raised diastolic pressures are transmitted to the pulmonary and systemic veins, and can cause pulmonary congestion and peripheral edema. Catecholamine activation may worsen coronary ischemia or induce cardiac arrhythmias. Activation of the renin–angiotensin system causes sodium and water retention and may promote further cardiovascular injury, including left ventricular hypertrophy and remodeling.

Diastolic Heart Failure

Diastolic HF occurs when there is reduced myocardial relaxation (e.g., from ischemia, myocyte hypertrophy, aging), increased passive stiffness of the ventricle (e.g., from infiltrative diseases such as hemochromatosis and amyloidosis), or limited ventricle mobility (e.g., from pericardial tamponade or extrinsic compression by tumor). In patients with left ventricular hypertrophy, ischemia may contribute to diastolic HF even when there are no significant coronary stenoses, because the elevated diastolic pressures may impair blood flow through capillaries and small resistance vessels.

Causes and Precipitants

The most common cause of HF is left ventricular systolic dysfunction, which typically results from coronary artery disease (Box 2-1). These patients may have a history of myocardial infarction or may have viable but underperfused myocardium. In patients with a history of HF, a frequent precipitant is dietary or fluid indiscretion or medication non-compliance. Tachyarrhythmias (most commonly atrial fibrillation) may reduce cardiac output by limiting the duration of ventricular filling, increasing myocardial oxygen demands, and eliminating "atrial kick." Atrial kick refers to atrial contraction, which promotes ventricular filling during diastole. Loss of atrial kick may precipitate HF in patients with stiffened ventricles from diastolic dysfunction. Myocardial infarction or ischemia can cause ventricular stiffening (diastolic dysfunction), reduced muscle mass for pumping blood, valvular leakage from papillary muscle dysfunction, and increased oxygen demand from pain and tachycardia, all of which may precipitate or contribute to HF. Systemic infections or hyperthyroidism increase the metabolic rate, which increases the workload on the heart. Newly prescribed medications may cause salt retention, myocardial depression, or arrhythmias (Table 2-1).

SYMPTOMS

1. Dyspnea, orthopnea (dyspnea upon lying supine), and paroxysmal nocturnal dyspnea are common symptoms of pulmonary congestion. Patients with paroxysmal nocturnal dyspnea describe wakening from sleep with shortness of breath. The presence and

Box 2-1. Common Precipitants of Heart Failure

Anemia

Dietary indiscretion

Hypertension

Hyperthyroidism

Infection, endocarditis

Medications (see Table 2-1)

Myocardial infarction

Myocarditis

Noncompliance with medications or fluid restriction

Pregnancy

Pulmonary embolism

Tachyarrhythmias or bradyarrhythmias

Adapted from Givertz MM, Colucci WS, Braunwald E. Clinical aspects of heart failure: pulmonary edema, high-output failure. In: Zipes DP, Libby P, Bonow RO, Braunwald E, editors. *Braunwald's Heart Disease: A Textbook of Cardiovascular Medicine*, 7th ed. Philadelphia. WB Saunders; 2005.

severity of orthopnea can be assessed by asking (a) "With how many pillows do you sleep?" and (b) "With how many pillows did you sleep weeks/months ago?" If there is an increase in the number of pillows, ask what symptoms prompted the change. When orthopnea is severe, patients may be unable to sleep in bed and may choose to sleep in a recliner or chair.

2. Fatigue, exercise intolerance, and mental obtundation are symptoms of poor cardiac output.
3. Peripheral edema suggests right-sided HF.
4. Weight gain results from fluid retention.

Table 2-1. Potentially Dangerous Medications in Patients with Heart Failure (HF)

Medication	Precaution	Time to Onset of HF	Recommendation
Glucocorticoids	Sodium and fluid retention	Days to weeks	Use lowest dose possible Monitor for heart failure symptoms
Nonsteroidal anti-inflammatory drugs	Sodium and fluid retention	Days to 1 month	Avoid in patients with symptomatic heart failure, if possible Use aspirin in patients with a history of or risk factors for cardiovascular disease
Class I and III anti-arrhythmics	Negative inotropic effects Pro-arrhythmic effects	Hours to months	Avoid all class I anti-arrhythmics Avoid class III ibutilide and sotalol Consider amiodarone or dofetilide if symptomatic or non-device-managed arrhythmias
Calcium channel blockers	Negative inotropic effects	2–3 months	Avoid verapamil, diltiazem, nifedipine, nisoldipine, nicardipine
Metformin	Lactic acidosis	Dependent on renal function	Avoid in class III or IV heart failure and in patients with a history of hospitalizations for heart failure

Continued

Table 2-1. Potentially Dangerous Medications in Patients with Heart Failure (HF)—cont'd

Medication	Precaution	Time to Onset of HF	Recommendation
Thiazolidinediones	Fluid retention	Within 8 weeks	Avoid in class III or class IV heart failure Monitor for heart failure symptoms
Cilostazol	Ventricular tachycardia and premature ventricular complexes	Unknown	Do not use in heart failure patients
Amphetamines	Tachycardia, arrhythmias, peripheral α and β agonists	Unknown	Do not use in heart failure patients
Carbamazepine	Proarrhythmic, negative inotrope and chromotrope	Unknown	Avoid, if possible
Clozapine	Unknown	Weeks to years	Monitor for heart failure symptoms
Tricyclic antidepressants	Negative inotropic effects Proarrhythmic effects	Weeks to years	Avoid, if possible
Beta-2-agonists	Positive chronotropic effects Hypokalemia promotes arrhythmias	Unknown	Use inhaled route and lowest dose as possible

Adapted from Amabile CM and Spencer AP. Keeping your patient with heart failure safe: A review of potentially dangerous medications, *Arch Int Med.* 2004;164:709–720.

SIGNS

The goal of the focused physical exam is to determine volume status and to search for potential precipitants of the HF.

1. Jugular Venous Distension

Jugular venous pressure (JVP), which reflects right atrial pressure (central venous pressure), is estimated by examining the internal jugular veins. We do not recommend using the external jugular vein pulsations to estimate central venous pressure, because valves in these veins may lead to inaccurate readings. To assess JVP, turn the patient's head slightly away from the side being examined and elevate the head of the bed to at least 30 degrees until the jugular venous pulsations are visible in the lower part of the neck. Several features help differentiate internal jugular pulsations from carotid pulsations. The internal jugular vein is not visible (lies deep to the sternocleidomastoid muscles), is rarely palpable, and the level of its pulsations drops with inspiration or as the patient becomes more upright.

The jugular vein pulsations usually have two elevations and two troughs. The first elevation (*a wave*) corresponds to the slight rise in atrial pressure resulting from atrial contraction. The first descent (*x descent*) reflects a fall in atrial pressure that starts with atrial relaxation. The second elevation (*v wave*) corresponds to ventricular systole when blood is entering the right atrium from the vena cavae while the tricuspid valve is closed. Finally, the second descent (*y descent*) reflects falling right atrial pressure as the tricuspid valve opens and blood drains from the atrium into the ventricle.

Once the highest point of internal jugular pulsation has been identified, the vertical distance between this point and the sternal angle represents the JVP. Regardless of the patient's position, the sternal angle remains approximately 5 cm above the right atrium. Venous pressure greater than 3 to 4 cm above the sternal notch is considered elevated, suggesting right-sided HF, constrictive pericarditis, tricuspid stenosis, or superior vena cava syndrome.

2. Heart

The heart examination should include assessment of the cardiac impulse (lateral displacement suggests cardiomegaly), heart rate (decompensated HF causes tachycardia), rhythm, murmurs (such as aortic stenosis or mitral regurgitation), and extra heart sounds (S_3 or S_4). An S_3 is a soft, low-frequency sound caused by vibrations of the ventricular walls, valves, and supporting structures as blood decelerates in the left ventricle during rapid ventricular filling. Although an S_3 is normal in some healthy children and young athletes, the presence of an S_3 in older adults suggests an abnormality, such as left HF or mitral regurgitation. The fourth heart sound (S_4) is caused by vibrations in the ventricular walls and supporting structures as blood from atrial contraction decelerates in the ventricle. An S_4 occurs when there is increased resistance to ventricular filling (diastolic dysfunction). A loud, widely split S_2 supports the diagnosis of pulmonary hypertension. Muffled heart sounds and a globular heart on chest x-ray suggest a pericardial effusion and should prompt assessment for *pulsus paradoxus* (more than 10 mmHg fall in systolic blood pressure with inspiration).

3. Lungs

a. Crackles

The crackles ("Velcro" sound) of HF are described as "wet" as compared to the "dry" crackles of pulmonary fibrosis, and are caused by air moving through fluid-filled airways. In mild HF, crackles will be limited to the lung bases. Atelectasis also causes bibasilar crackles, but the crackles of atelectasis clear after several repeated inspirations. Crackles will be detected higher in the chest with worsening severity of HF. Crackles may be absent in patients with chronic HF even in the setting of elevated pulmonary capillary wedge pressure. Also, crackles may be difficult to hear in patients with emphysema or other coexisting pulmonary diseases.

b. Pleural Effusion

Pleural effusions in patients with HF usually do not require thoracentesis, and typically resolve with diuresis. Although effusions are classically transudative, diuretic therapy can cause the effusion to become exudative. In this setting, the traditional Light's criteria used to differentiate transudative from exudative pleural effusions may be misleading and it may be more appropriate to use the pleural fluid/serum albumin gradient. A gradient >1.2 g/dL suggests that the effusion is likely due to HF.

c. Wheezing

Some patients with pulmonary edema develop wheezing. Potential mechanisms include reflex bronchoconstriction from elevation of pulmonary or bronchial vascular pressure, and decreased airway size from intraluminal edema and bronchial mucosal swelling.

4. Pitting Edema

Right-sided HF reduces venous return to the heart and causes pitting edema of the lower extremities. Because gravity plays an important role in the formation of edema, patients who are predominantly bed-bound may have very little lower extremity edema even when there is profound fluid overload. In these cases, the pitting edema may be detected at the sacrum or along the lower back. Peripheral edema may be absent in patients with chronic HF.

5. Cheyne-Stokes Respiration

Cheyne-Stokes respiration is a breathing disorder of sleep seen in almost one-half of HF patients with ejection fractions below 40%. Cheyne-Stokes breathing is characterized by a crescendo–decrescendo alteration in tidal volume separated by periods of apnea or hypopnea. The mechanisms for Cheyne-Stokes respiration are not fully understood, but may include increased central nervous system sensitivity to changes in arterial partial pressures of oxygen and carbon dioxide. Therapeutic options include medical optimization of HF, nocturnal oxygen therapy, and nasal continuous positive airway pressure.

6. Other Findings

Other findings of right-sided HF include hepatosplenomegaly, ascites, and imaging evidence of bowel wall edema (which may affect medication absorption). Other findings of left-sided HF and poor cardiac output include mental obtundation, cool skin, and cachexia.

LABORATORY DATA

Initial laboratory testing should include:

1. Electrolytes, blood urea nitrogen, creatinine, and complete blood count (with differential if infection is suspected)

2. PA and lateral chest x-ray

Classic chest x-ray findings of HF include:

a) Cardiomegaly—defined on chest x-ray as a "cardiothoracic ratio" (horizontal width of the

heart divided by the widest internal diameter of the thorax) above 0.5
b) Large hila with indistinct vessel margins
c) Cephalization of flow—present when upper lobe vessels in an upright patient are larger than the lower lobe vessels at approximately the same distance from the hilum (normally, the upper lobe vessels are smaller than the lower lobe vessels because gravity directs most blood flow to the lung bases). Cephalization of flow implies elevated left heart pressures.
d) Pleural effusions
e) Kerley B lines—imply interstitial edema and occur when fluid thickens the interlobular septa, causing short lines to appear perpendicular to the pleural surface
f) Alveolar edema
g) Peribronchial cuffing—develops when fluid extravasates from peri-bronchial vessels and outlines the bronchi. The bronchi appear as dark circles surrounded by a water-dense ring.
h) Fluid in the interlobar fissures

Many of these findings may be obscured or distorted if there is underlying lung disease. Findings may be absent in patients with chronic HF who have longstanding elevations in pulmonary capillary wedge pressure

3. Electrocardiography

Electrocardiography (ECG) may demonstrate abnormal cardiac rhythm, ischemia, prior evidence of myocardial infarction, or left ventricular hypertrophy.

4. B-type Natriuretic Peptide

B-type natriuretic peptide (BNP) is primarily produced in the ventricles in response to ventricular strain or stretch. This hormone has shown initial promise in rapidly differentiating HF from lung disease in patients presenting to the emergency department with acute dyspnea. BNP levels <50 pg/mL may have a negative predictive value for HF as high as 96% (i.e., the probability of not having HF given a BNP <50 pg/ml is 96%). Therefore, HF is an unlikely cause of dyspnea in an untreated patient with normal BNP levels, and echocardiography may be unnecessary in this setting.

5. Echocardiography

Findings on history, physical examination, the ECG, and chest x-ray occur with similar frequencies in both systolic and diastolic HF. Therefore, these symptoms and signs cannot be used to reliably differentiate systolic HF from diastolic HF. For this reason, two-dimensional, M-mode echocardiography should be obtained in all patients presenting with HF unless this test has been performed recently and there has been no interval change in the patient's medical history. Echocardiography provides useful information about the left ventricular ejection fraction, valvular dysfunction, regional wall motion abnormalities, ventricular hypertrophy, pericardial disease, and pulmonary hypertension. Echocardiography may also diagnose a dilated (4-chamber enlargement) or restrictive ("starry sky") cardiomyopathy or diastolic dysfunction.

    Echocardiographic evidence for diastolic HF includes normal systolic function and reversal of the "E to A" ratio. The E wave refers to the peak velocity of blood flow across the mitral valve during *early* diastolic filling. The A wave corresponds to peak velocity of blood flow across the mitral valve during *atrial* contraction. Normally, the E-wave velocity is greater than the A-wave velocity, and the E to A ratio is approximately 1.5. In early diastolic dysfunction, the stiff heart relaxes slowly. In this setting, atrial contraction contributes relatively more to ventricular filling and there is reversal of the E to A ratio (<1.0). In patients with severe diastolic dysfunction, the very high end-diastolic left ventricular pressures significantly limit the contribution of atrial contraction to left ventricular filling and the E to A ratio rises again, often to greater than 2.0.

CARDIAC CATHETERIZATION

Cardiac catheterization is usually performed when there is no obvious cause for the HF or when myocardial ischemia is suspected (for example, when patients describe angina or if there is objective evidence of myocardial infarction). Cardiac catheterization can also demonstrate impaired ventricular relaxation and filling by providing a direct measurement of ventricular diastolic pressure.

TREATMENT (Table 2-2)

While initiating drug therapy, potential precipitants of the HF should be identified and treated.

Medications (Table 2-3)

1. Diuretics

Diuretics are an important early component of treatment for patients with volume overload. Patients with right-sided HF often have bowel wall edema, which may limit intestinal absorption of oral medication. Therefore, it is appropriate to initiate treatment with an intravenous loop diuretic. Furosemide is the first-line agent unless there is a severe sulfa allergy. The weaker diuretic, ethacrynic acid, should be substituted if there is a contraindication to furosemide. Patients who are furosemide-naive should receive furosemide 10–40 mg intravenously (IV), with the initial dose depending on the severity of symptoms and the desired rapidity of effect.

Continued on p. 44

Table 2-2. Controlled Trials of Medications for the Treatment of Symptomatic Systolic Heart Failure

Trial and Year Published	Trial Size	Severity of Heart Failure	Estimated First-Year Mortality in Control Group	Background Treatment in at Least One Third of Patients	Treatment Added	Trial Duration (years)	Primary Endpoint	Relative Risk Reduction (%) in Primary Endpoint
ACE Inhibitors								
CONSENSUS 1987	253	End-stage	52	Spironolactone	Enalapril 20 mg twice daily	0.54	Death	40
SOLVD-T 1991	2569	Mild to severe	15.7	None	Enalapril 10 mg twice daily	3.5	Death	16

Beta-Blockers

Trial								
CIBIS-2 1999	2647	Moderate to severe	13.2	ACE inhibitor	Bisoprolol 10 mg once daily	1.3	Death	34
MERIT-HF 1999	3991	Mild to severe	11	ACE inhibitor	Metoprolol CR/XL 200 mg once daily	1	Death	34
COPERNICUS 2001	2289	Severe	19.7	ACE inhibitor	Carvedilol 25 mg twice daily	0.87	Death	35
Angiotensin Receptor Blockers								
Val-HeFT 2001	5010	Mild to severe	8	ACE inhibitor	Valsartan 160 mg twice daily	1.9	Death or morbidity	13

Continued

Table 2-2. Controlled Trials of Medications for the Treatment of Symptomatic Systolic Heart Failure—cont'd

Trial and Year Published	Trial Size	Severity of Heart Failure	Estimated First-Year Mortality in Control Group	Background Treatment in at Least One Third of Patients	Treatment Added	Trial Duration (years)	Primary Endpoint	Relative Risk Reduction (%) in Primary Endpoint
CHARM-Alternative 2003	2028	Mild to severe	12.6	Beta-blocker	Candesartan 32 mg once daily	2.8	Cardiovascular death or hospital admission for heart failure	23
CHARM-Added 2003	2548	Moderate to severe	10.6	ACE inhibitor + beta-blocker	Candesartan 32 mg once daily	3.4	Cardiovascular death or hospital admission for heart failure	15

Aldosterone Blockade

RALES 1999	1663	Severe	25	ACE inhibitor	Spironolactone 25–50 mg once daily	2	Death	30

Hydralazine and Isosorbide Dinitrate

V-HeFT-1 1986	459	Mild to severe	26.4	—	Hydralazine 75 mg three or four times daily; isosorbide dinitrate 40 mg four times daily	2.3	Death	34

Continued

Table 2-2. Controlled Trials of Medications for the Treatment of Symptomatic Systolic Heart Failure—cont'd

Trial and Year Published	Trial Size	Severity of Heart Failure	Estimated First-Year Mortality in Control Group	Background Treatment in at Least One Third of Patients	Treatment Added	Trial Duration (years)	Primary Endpoint	Relative Risk Reduction (%) in Primary Endpoint
				Digitalis Glycosides				
DIG 1997	6800	Mild to severe	11	ACE-I	Digoxin	3.1	Death	0

Adapted with permission from McMurray JJV, Pfeffer MA. Heart failure. *Lancet* 2005;365:1877–1889.

Table 2-3. Medications for Treating Heart Failure

Medication Class	Comments
Diuretics	Use early in the course of treatment. Use intravenous route initially.
Angiotensin-converting enzyme (ACE) inhibitors	Monitor for hyperkalemia. Use with caution if there is coexisting renal insufficiency. May cause cough. Preferred over angiotensin receptor blockers (ARBs).
Angiotensin receptor blockers	Monitor for hyperkalemia. Use with caution if there is coexisting renal insufficiency. Do not cause cough.
Beta-blockers	Start with low dose and titrate slowly. Do not initiate in the setting of acute heart failure. Reduce the beta-blocker dose during a heart failure exacerbation.
Digoxin	Improves symptoms and reduces hospitalizations but does not reduce mortality.
Aldosterone antagonists	Monitor for hyperkalemia. Eplerenone has fewer side effects than spironolactone (gynecomastia).
Hydralazine and nitrates	Reduce mortality but effect is not as large as for ACE inhibitors. Use only if patient is intolerant of ACE inhibitors and ARBs.

Patients who chronically use oral furosemide can be given an IV dose that is the same or slightly higher than their usual daily dose. Short-term response (hours) to the diuretic is assessed by monitoring the patient's symptoms and measuring urine output. Catheterization of the bladder is appropriate for patients who are unable to accurately collect their urine because of physical or mental constraints. If urine output is suboptimal, the furosemide dose should be doubled (10–20–40–80–160 mg), but no more than 200 mg IV furosemide should be given at any one time because of the risk of ototoxicity. If urine output remains suboptimal on the maximal dose of furosemide but the patient remains volume overloaded, chlorothiazide or metolazone can be added. For example, chlorothiazide 250 mg IV can be given 30 to 60 minutes before a dose of furosemide 200 mg IV. However, these combinations should be used with caution because of the risk of severe hypokalemia, and the serum potassium concentration should be monitored closely. If this combination regimen fails, continuous IV furosemide can be infused at a rate of 0.5 to 30 mg/hr. A loading dose of 200 mg IV furosemide should be given upon initiation of the continuous infusion.

To improve the efficacy of the diuretic, dietary salt intake should be limited to 2 g/day and fluid intake should be limited to 2 L/day. If possible, the patient should be weighed daily on the same scale and "In's and Out's" (I/Os) should be meticulously recorded. Diuretics are dosed to achieve a daily I/O goal or weight, which should be determined by the medical team based on the volume status from physical examination and on laboratory data, such as blood urea nitrogen and serum creatinine measurements. Typical I/O goals are −2 L, −1 L, −500 mL, "even" (fluid intake = fluid loss), + 500 mL, + 1 L. Serum potassium concentrations should be monitored at least daily (more often with aggressive diuresis) and repleted with consideration of the underlying renal function. When the patient is ready for transition from IV to oral furosemide, the oral dose should be about one half the IV dose.

2. Angiotensin-converting enzyme inhibitors

Angiotensin-converting enzyme (ACE) inhibitors improve mortality, symptoms of HF, left ventricular ejection fraction, and exercise tolerance and reduce hospitalizations. ACE inhibitors should be initiated early during the treatment of HF before excessive diuresis has occurred. In hospitalized settings, especially when patients are ACE-inhibitor naive, ACE inhibitors with short half-lives, such as captopril, are often used so that dosages can be rapidly titrated as needed. For example, captopril, which is dosed three times daily, can be initiated at 6.25 mg and increased by 6.25 mg increments with each successive dose, as tolerated by blood pressure. Although a medication like captopril is easy to titrate in the hospital, patients should be discharged on once-daily medications to improve compliance, especially since they will likely be taking several other medications. As a rough rule, captopril 12.5 mg three times daily is interchangeable with lisinopril 5 mg daily; captopril 25 mg three times daily is interchangeable with lisinopril 10 mg daily; and captopril 50 mg three times daily is interchangeable with lisinopril 20 mg daily.

ACE inhibitors can increase serum creatinine measurements, but levels usually stabilize in 2 to 4 weeks. One recommended approach is to stop the ACE inhibitor or reduce the dose if the serum creatinine rises 30% above baseline values and/or the serum potassium exceeds 5.0 mEq/L.

Although angiotensin-receptor blockers (ARBs) do not activate the bradykinin system (and are, therefore, unlikely to produce cough), these medications probably have the same risk of hyperkalemia and renal insufficiency as the ACE inhibitors. Because there are extensive placebo-controlled data showing the benefit of ACE inhibitors in HF, these medications should be first-line therapy. ARBs are the next appropriate choice for patients who cannot tolerate ACE inhibitors (cough, angioedema). If renal insufficiency or hyperkalemia are limiting factors, then hydralazine and isosorbide dinitrate should be substituted (combination hydralazine and isosorbide dinitrate was the first treatment shown to reduce mortality in HF, but this combination was subsequently shown to be less effective than ACE inhibition).

3. Beta-adrenergic blockers

In earlier years, beta-blockers were contraindicated in HF because of their negative inotropic effects. However, three beta-blockers (carvedilol, long-acting metoprolol, and bisoprolol) have subsequently been shown to improve morbidity and mortality in patients with HF. Beta-blockers probably exert beneficial effects by reducing arrhythmias, ischemia, and myocardial consumption (reduced heart rate), and by counteracting the detrimental effects of an activated sympathetic nervous system. These medications should be initiated only after the patient's condition has stabilized and the volume status has normalized. Dosages should be titrated over weeks until the target dose is reached or side effects (bradycardia, hypotension) develop. Doses should be reduced in patients presenting with severe HF.

4. Digoxin

Digoxin reduces hospitalization, improves symptoms and quality of life, but does not lower mortality in patients with HF. Therefore, digoxin is an appropriate agent to add if the patient remains symptomatic despite optimal medical therapy or requires frequent hospitalizations for HF.

5. Mineralocorticoid receptor antagonists

The mineralocorticoid receptor (MR) antagonists, spironolactone and eplerenone, appear to reduce the risk of death and hospitalization in sick HF patients who are already receiving ACE inhibitor therapy. However, there is concern for dangerous hyperkalemia with combination ACE inhibitor and MR antagonist therapy, especially because many HF patients have reduced renal function. Therefore, some authorities recommend avoiding MR antagonists until further studies have been completed.

Medical Therapy for Diastolic Heart Failure

Clinical trials testing medications for the treatment of diastolic HF are limited. ACE inhibitors and ARBs may improve exercise capacity and reduce hospitalizations for diastolic HF. Diuretics are appropriate for volume management, but these medications should be used with caution because patients with diastolic dysfunction are sensitive to excessive preload reduction. In patients with diastolic dysfunction and atrial fibrillation or other tachyarrhythmias, beta-blockers or non-dihydropyridine calcium channel blockers can be used to slow the heart rate and lengthen diastole so that the ventricle has a longer filling time.

Hospital Discharge Instructions

Prior to hospital discharge, patients should be educated about dietary salt and fluid restriction and should be instructed to weigh themselves daily on the same scale. The home furosemide dose should be doubled if the weight increases by 2 lb over the course of 1 day. The patient should call his/her physician if the weight increases by ≥ 5 lb or if clinical signs develop, such as a change in the number of pillows needed to sleep, reduced exercise tolerance, or peripheral edema.

REFERENCES

Review Articles and Textbooks

1. Jessup M, Brozena S. Heart failure. *N Engl J Med*. 2003;348:2007–2018.
2. Angeja BG, Grossman W. Evaluation and management of diastolic heart failure. *Circulation* 2003;107:659–663.
3. Zile M, Brutsaert D. New concepts in diastolic dysfunction and diastolic heart failure: Part I: Diagnosis, prognosis, and measurements of diastolic function. *Circulation* 2002;105:1387–1393.
4. Colucci WS, Braunwald E. In: Braunwald E, Zipes DP, Libby P, editors. *Heart Disease: A Textbook of Cardiovascular Medicine*, 6th ed. Philadelphia. WB Saunders Company; 2001.
5. Quaranta AJ, D'Alonzo GE, Krachman SL. Cheyne-Stokes respiration during sleep in congestive heart failure. *Chest* 1997;111:467–473.
6. Aurigemma GP, Gaasch WH. Diastolic heart failure. *N Engl J Med*. 2004;351:1097–1105.
7. McMurray JJV, Pfeffer MA. Heart failure. *Lancet* 2005;365:1877–1889.

Diagnosis

1. Bickley LS, Szilagyi PG. *A Guide to Physical Examination and History Taking*, 9th ed. Philadelphia. Lippincott, Williams & Wilkins; 1995.

2. Gehlbach BK, Geppert E. The pulmonary manifestations of left heart failure. *Chest* 2004;125:669–682.

3. de Denus S, Pharand C, Williamson DR. Brain natriuretic peptide in the management of heart failure: The versatile neurohormone. *Chest* 2004;125:652–668.

4. Wang CS, FitzGerald JM, Schulzer M, et al. Does this dyspneic patient in the emergency department have congestive heart failure? *JAMA* 2005;294:1944–1956.

Treatment

1. Amabile CM, Spencer AP. Keeping your patient with heart failure safe: A review of potentially dangerous medications. *Arch Intern Med*. 2004;164:709–720.

2. Gomberg-Maitland M, Baran DA, Fuster V. Treatment of congestive heart failure: guidelines for the primary care physician and the heart failure specialist. *Arch Intern Med*. 2001;161:342–352.

3. Konstam MA, Mann DL. Contemporary medical options for treating patients with heart failure. *Circulation* 2002;105:2244–2246.

4. Hunt SA, Baker DW, Chin MH, et al. ACC/AHA Guidelines for the evaluation and management of chronic heart failure in the adult: Executive summary a report of the American College of Cardiology/American Heart Association task force on practice guidelines (committee to revise the 1995 guidelines for the evaluation and management of heart failure). *Circulation* 2001;104:2996–3007.

5. Foody JM, Farrell MH, Krumholz HM. β-blocker therapy in heart failure: Scientific review. *JAMA* 2002;287:883–889.

6. Rahimtoola SH. Digitalis therapy for patients in clinical heart failure. *Circulation* 2004;109: 2942–2946.
7. Brater DC. Diuretic therapy. *N Engl J Med*. 1998;339:387–395.

Unstable Angina and Non-ST Elevation Myocardial Infarction

KEY POINTS

1. Unstable angina and non-ST elevation myocardial infarction are usually caused by non-occluding thrombus forming on a ruptured plaque in a coronary artery.

2. Initial evaluation and management should include a complete blood count (CBC), serum chemistries, cardiac injury markers (troponin I, troponin T, or MB fraction of creatine kinase [CK-MB]), 12-lead electrocardiogram (EKG), telemetry, and IV access. History and physical examination should assess for complications such as hemodynamic instability or hypoxemia, and determine the level of risk for adverse outcomes.

3. Anti-ischemic therapy with nitroglycerin (NTG), beta-blockers, morphine, and oxygen should be initiated in all patients.

4. Aspirin, unfractionated or low molecular weight heparin, and clopidogrel should be initiated in the absence of contraindications. If cardiac angiography is planned, administration of clopidogrel may be deferred until a decision is made regarding the need for coronary artery bypass grafting (CABG).

5. Eptifibatide or tirofiban (GP IIb/IIIa inhibitors) should be initiated in patients with high-risk features, ongoing ischemia, elevated cardiac injury markers, or significant

ST segment or T-wave changes. GP IIb/IIIa inhibitors should also be used if the patient will undergo cardiac angiography.

6. Patients at intermediate or high risk of adverse outcomes should undergo early coronary angiography and revascularization.

DEFINITIONS

The following terms have been defined by the American College of Cardiology (ACC) and the American Heart Association (AHA). Acute coronary syndrome (ACS) refers to a collection of symptoms that are consistent with acute myocardial ischemia, and includes unstable angina (UA), non-ST-elevation myocardial infarction (NSTEMI), and ST-elevation myocardial infarction (STEMI). These conditions lie on a continuum of severity.

NSTEMI: Ischemia resulting in myocardial damage, with detectable markers of myocardial injury, including the MB fraction of creatine kinase (CK-MB), troponin I (cTnI), or troponin T (cTnT), but no ST-elevation on the electrocardiogram (EKG).

UA: Myocardial ischemia without detectable markers of myocardial injury. Because cardiac injury markers are not immediately available, the distinction between UA and NSTEMI may not be made with certainty on initial presentation.

EPIDEMIOLOGY

Coronary artery disease (CAD) is the leading cause of death in the United States. UA and NSTEMI account for over 5 million emergency department visits and over 1 million admissions per year. Most deaths from UA or NSTEMI are due to sudden death or acute myocardial infarction (AMI).

PATHOGENESIS

Potential Mechanisms

UA and NSTEMI occur when there is a relative deficit in myocardial oxygen delivery. This may be due to increased myocardial oxygen demand or decreased oxygen supply. The major causes of UA and NSTEMI are described in the following text:

- Non-occluding thrombus forming on a ruptured plaque—most common cause of UA and NSTEMI. Subsequent embolization of platelet or plaque particles may result in release of cardiac injury markers
- Coronary artery spasm (Prinzmetal's angina)—results in flow obstruction and may lead to UA and NSTEMI
- Progressive coronary artery narrowing from atherosclerosis or restenosis after cardiac revascularization
- Arterial inflammation—may lead to narrowing of coronary arteries, plaque rupture, and stenosis
- Secondary UA—cause of oxygen imbalance is outside of the coronary circulation. Potential causes include:
  - Increase in myocardial oxygen demand from fever and tachycardia
  - Decrease in myocardial oxygen supply from hypotension or hypoxia

CLINICAL FEATURES

Introduction

Patients with UA may present with any of the following three scenarios:

- Rest angina—angina at rest lasting at least 20 minutes. May also occur in patients with NSTEMI
- Increasing angina—existing angina that has been increasing in frequency, duration, or intensity. The intensity should be increased by at least one classification to at least Class 3 (angina occurring after walking 1 to 2 level blocks or climbing 1 flight of stairs)
- New onset angina—newly diagnosed angina of at least Class 3 intensity (see preceding text)

Initial Evaluation and Probability of ACS

The evaluation of UA and NSTEMI involves two major steps. The first step is to determine whether the patient is experiencing ACS. The second step is to determine the patient's risk of an adverse outcome. Aside from a thorough history and physical examination, an EKG and cardiac injury markers (CK with MB fraction, troponin I, or troponin T) should be obtained in persons with possible ACS.

According to the ACC/AHA Guidelines, the possibility that a constellation of signs and symptoms are due to ACS may be stratified as follows:

- High likelihood of ACS:
  - History of chest or left arm pain or discomfort, or occurrence of prior angina equivalent. History of myocardial infarction or CAD
  - Physical examination findings of hypotension, diaphoresis, pulmonary edema, rales, or transient mitral regurgitation
  - EKG findings of new and transient ST segment changes > 0.05 mV or T wave inversion > 0.2 mV associated with symptoms
  - Elevations of cardiac injury markers
- Intermediate likelihood of ACS: No findings within high likelihood category, and

- History of chest or left arm pain or discomfort as primary complaint, age > 70 years old, male sex, or history of diabetes mellitus
- Physical examination suggestive of vascular disease outside the coronary arteries
- EKG findings of fixed Q waves, abnormal but not new ST-segment or T wave changes
- Normal levels of cardiac injury markers
- Low likelihood of ACS: No findings within the high or intermediate likelihood category, and
  - History that may be consistent with myocardial ischemia or recent cocaine use
  - Physical examination of chest discomfort reproduced by manual compression or palpation
  - EKG findings of flattened or inverted T-waves in leads with dominant R waves or normal EKG
  - Normal levels of cardiac injury markers

History

Aside from the sex and age of the patient, the history should focus on the patient's symptoms and presence of risk factors, including history of CAD. Typical angina is pain, pressure, or discomfort located in the chest or arm that reliably occurs with physical activity or emotional stress, and is relieved with rest or sublingual nitroglycerin. Some patients may have other symptoms, such as jaw, neck, epigastric, or upper extremity discomfort or pain that has a clear association with activity or stress; such events may be considered anginal equivalents. Elderly patients and patients with diabetes mellitus may present with atypical symptoms of angina, including new onset dyspnea on exertion, fatigue, or diaphoresis. History findings of older age, male sex, chest or left upper extremity discomfort, or pain are most consistent with acute cardiac ischemia.

Pleuritic chest pain, lower abdominal pain, well-localized chest pain, or fleeting pain lasting a few seconds is not consistent with angina.

However, presence of these symptoms does not necessarily exclude ACS. Up to 22% of patients with stabbing chest pain may be diagnosed with acute ischemia.

A history of myocardial infarction and older age results in a higher risk of severe or multi-vessel CAD. Diabetes mellitus and hypertension increase the risk of adverse outcomes.

PHYSICAL EXAMINATION

The physical examination should focus on determining:

- Whether other diagnoses may explain the patient's chest pain
- Whether other factors may be exacerbating the patient's condition (i.e., anemia, hyperthyroidism, hypoxemia)
- Whether significant hemodynamic compromise has occurred

Vital signs, including blood pressure in each arm, heart rate, respiratory rate, and oxygen saturation, should be determined.

Findings that suggest severe disease or increased risk of adverse outcomes include new-onset mitral regurgitation or evidence of left ventricular dysfunction (pulmonary crackles, S_3 gallop). The presence of cardiogenic shock portends high mortality rates of up to 60% and should be treated as a medical emergency.

Electrocardiogram

A 12-lead EKG should be obtained while the patient is symptomatic. ST segment deviation > 0.05 mV or T-wave inversions greater than 0.2 mV during an episode of angina that resolve when the patient is asymptomatic is highly suggestive of ACS. Continuous 12-lead EKG monitoring may also be performed. Patients with suspected or documented ACS should be observed with telemetry monitoring.

Box 3-1 lists the non-ACS causes of ST segment and T wave changes.

Cardiac Injury Markers

Cardiac injury markers should be obtained on presentation and every 8 hours for the first 24 hours. Often, an EKG is performed at the same time.

Troponins

Troponin I and Troponin T are markers of cardiac injury. Troponins are more specific and sensitive than CK for the diagnosis of myocardial infarction and may also allow for risk-stratification. Troponins are useful for diagnosis of recent myocardial infarction within 2 weeks of onset that may otherwise be missed by creatine kinase assays. Due to their increased sensitivity,

Box 3-1. Some Non-ACS Causes of ST-Segment and T-Wave Changes

ST segment depression

Left ventricular hypertrophy

Digoxin effect

ST segment elevation

Ventricular aneurysm

Pericarditis

Prinzmetal's angina

Early repolarization

Persistent juvenile pattern

Wolff-Parkinson-White syndrome

T-wave inversions

Left ventricular hypertrophy

CNS disease

Tricyclic antidepressants

troponins may also be elevated when CK–MB levels are normal, allowing for detection of "micro-infarctions."

Troponin levels correlate with the risk of death in patients with ACS. Patients with normal EKG findings and CK–MB levels but with elevated troponin levels have a higher risk of death than do patients with normal troponin levels. Patients with increased troponin levels may also benefit from more aggressive anti-platelet and anti-coagulation therapy.

Creatine Kinase

Measurement of CK–MB has traditionally been used in the diagnosis of myocardial injury. CK-MB is superior to troponins for early diagnosis of myocardial infarction, but it has lower sensitivity for the diagnosis of myocardial infarction > 36 hours after the event. CK-MB has a shorter half-life than troponins, which may be useful for the diagnosis of recurrent myocardial infarction.

Early Risk Stratification

Early risk-stratification (for short-term risk of death or non-fatal MI) allows identification of patients who may benefit from more aggressive anti-platelet and anti-coagulation therapy and early angiography. Two systems will be described here. The ACC/AHA Guidelines from 2002 allow risk-stratification based on history, physical examination and EKG findings, and cardiac marker levels. The Thrombolysis in MI (TIMI) risk score was developed and validated based on data from large clinical trials. It uses seven clinical variables to stratify patients into high-, medium-, and low-risk categories (Box 3-2).

MANAGEMENT

Overview

The management of suspected UA or NSTEMI involves:

Box 3-2. Early Risk Stratification in UA/NSTEMI

High Risk: At least one of the following:

- History of accelerating angina or ischemic symptoms within the preceding 48 hr
- Current episode of angina at rest lasting more than 20 min
- Clinical findings
  - Pulmonary edema (usually due to ischemia)
  - New or increasing murmur of mitral regurgitation
  - S_3 gallop
  - Hypotension, bradycardia, or tachycardia
  - Age greater than 75 years
- Electrocardiographic findings
  - Transient ST segment changes > 0.05 mV associated with rest angina
  - New bundle branch block
  - Sustained ventricular tachycardia
  - Elevated cardiac injury markers: Troponin I or T > 0.1 ng/mL

Intermediate Risk: Absence of high-risk findings and at least one of the following:

- History of myocardial infarction or coronary artery bypass graft (CABG), aspirin use, or peripheral or cerebrovascular disease
- Angina
  - At rest that is relieved with nitroglycerin, lasting less than 20 min
  - Recent episode of rest angina lasting longer than 20 min in a patient with at least a moderate risk of having CAD
- Age greater than 70 years
- Electrocardiographic findings
  - Inverted T-waves > 0.2 mV
    - Pathological Q waves
    - Slightly increased cardiac injury markers

Continued

Box 3-2. Early Risk Stratification in UA/NSTEMI—cont'd

Low Risk: Absence of high or intermediate risk findings and any of the following:

- New or worsening angina (at least Class III) within 2 weeks (pain lasting more than 20 min without prolonged rest in a patient with at least a moderate risk of having CAD)
- Electrocardiogram that is normal or without any acute changes
- Normal cardiac injury markers

TIMI Risk Score

Data from the TIMI 11B and ESSENCE trials were used to develop a scoring system to determine the risk of death, infarction, re-infarction, or recurrent ischemia requiring revascularization. For the TIMI risk score, seven variables are used. A numerical value of 1 is given if the variable is present and 0 if it is absent:

- Age 65 or older
- At least three risk factors for CAD present
- Prior angiographic coronary obstruction > 50%
- ST segment deviation on admission
- Two or more episodes of angina within the last 24 hours
- Elevated cardiac injury markers
- Use of aspirin within the previous week

A score if 0–2 is low risk, 3–4 is intermediate risk, and 5–7 is high risk.

From Braunwald E, Antman EM, Beasley JW, et al. ACC/AHA 2002 guideline update for the management of patients with unstable angina and non-ST-segment elevation myocardial infarction: a report of the American College of Cardiology/ American Heart Association Task Force on Practice Guidelines (Committee on the Management of Patients with Unstable Angina). 2002. Available at: http://www.acc.org/clinical/guide-lines/unstable/unstable.pdf.

- Performing initial stabilization and evaluation
- Determining the probability that the patient has an ACS
- Performing early risk stratification to determine the patient's short-term probability of death or non-fatal MI
- Initiating treatment
  - Anti-ischemic therapy
  - Anti-platelet therapy
  - Anti-coagulation
- Deciding whether a conservative medical or early invasive strategy is appropriate

Contrary to the management of STEMI, thrombolytic agents should not be used in patients with UA/NSTEMI, because the majority of these patients do not have occlusion of the coronary arteries. See Table 3-1 for commonly used medications in UA/NSTEMI.

Initial Stabilization and Evaluation

Patients with UA/NSTEMI should have a history, physical examination, cardiac injury markers, and EKG performed as described above. Laboratory testing in addition to cardiac markers should include a complete blood count (CBC), coagulation panel (prothrombin time, International Normalized Ratio, activated partial thromboplastin time), serum chemistries (electrolytes, magnesium), serum glucose, lipid profile, blood urea nitrogen, and creatinine.

Intravenous access should be established. Aspirin at a dose of 162 to 325 mg should be administered and chewed by the patient for faster absorption. Nitroglycerin (NTG) should be given for pain control at a dose of 0.4 mg sublingually every 5 minutes as needed, up to three doses. Intravenous morphine sulfate (1–5 mg initially, followed by 2–8 mg every 10 minutes) may be given for persistent pain or discomfort not relieved with NTG. Oxygen delivery

Table 3-1. Therapy for Unstable Angina and Non ST-elevation Myocardial Infarction

	Dose	Major adverse reactions	Contraindications/Cautions
Nitroglycerin	0.4 mg sublingual or spray every 5 min for 3 doses 10 µg/min continuous IV infusion. May increase by 10 µg/min every 5 min to a maximum rate of 200 µg/min	Headaches Hypotension Methemoglobinemia (rare)	Do not use if patient has taken a phosphodiesterase inhibitor for sexual dysfunction (e.g., sildenafil) within 24 hours. Patients also should not take a phosphodiesterase inhibitor within 24 hours of NTG use Use with caution in patients at risk for severe hypotension, such as those with right ventricular infarction or severe aortic stenosis

Morphine Sulfate	1–5 mg IV, may be repeated every 10 min as needed	Hypotension Respiratory depression Nausea, vomiting May be reversed with naloxone 0.4–2.0 mg IV	
Beta-blockers Metoprolol	5 mg IV over 2 min. Repeat every 5 min for a total of 15 mg as tolerated 15 min after last IV dose, start 25–50 mg orally every 6 hr × 48 hr Maintenance dosing of 50–200 mg orally twice a day	Hypotension Reactive airways exacerbation Worsening of heart failure	Bradycardia, severe first-degree, or any second- or third-degree AV block Reactive airways disease
Atenolol	5 mg IV and repeated in 5 min as tolerated 1–2 hr after the last IV dose, initiate 50–100 mg orally per day		

Continued

Table 3-1. Therapy for Unstable Angina and Non ST-elevation Myocardial Infarction—cont'd

	Dose	Major adverse reactions	Contraindications/Cautions
Propanolol	Maintenance dosing of 50–200 mg orally daily 0.5–1.0 mg IV 1–2 hr after the last IV dose, initiate 40–80 mg orally every 6–8 hr Maintenance dosing of 20–80 mg orally twice a day		
Esmolol	0.1 mg/kg/min continuous IV infusion Increase by 0.05 mg/kg/min every 10–15 min as tolerated, to a maximum dose of 0.3 mg/kg/min		
Calcium Channel Blockers		Hypotension, bradycardia, worsening, heart failure	Congestive heart failure or pulmonary edema

Verapamil	80–160 mg orally three times daily (120–480 mg orally daily if slow-release formulation)	Bradycardia, heart block
Diltiazem	30–80 mg orally four times daily (120–320 mg orally daily if slow-release formulation)	
Aspirin	Initial dose of 162–325 mg chewed orally	Gastritis, gastrointestinal ulcers, abdominal pain	Should not be used in patients with significant active bleeding
	Maintenance does of 81–162 mg orally daily	Bleeding May trigger asthma	Should not be used in patients with hypersensitivity to aspirin, or in patients with aspirin-induced asthma
Clopidogrel	Initial loading dose of 300 mg orally Maintenance dose of 75 mg orally daily	Bleeding Rare cases of thrombotic thrombocytopenic purpura and neutropenia Rash Diarrhea	Patients with active bleeding should not receive clopidogrel

should be started. Bed rest with continuous ECG monitoring should be initiated.

Early risk-stratification methods have already been described. Risk stratification is essential in guiding subsequent therapy, including choice of anti-platelet therapy and initiation of an early invasive strategy.

Anti-Ischemic Therapy

Nitroglycerin, beta-blockers, and morphine sulfate are the mainstays of anti-ischemic therapy. Other adjunctive medications include nondihydropyridine calcium channel blockers (verapamil and diltiazem), angiotensin converting enzyme inhibitors (ACE-I), and oxygen.

Nitroglycerin

Nitroglycerin (NTG) in either sublingual (SL) or spray form should be used for relief of angina and ischemia (ACC/AHA Class I indication; see reference for details on ACC/AHA indication classification). NTG 0.4 mg SL or spray may be given every 5 minutes for a total of three doses. If pain persists, NTG 10 μg/min continuous intravenous infusion should be started. The rate may be increased by 10 μg/min every 5 minutes until a maximum rate of 200 μg/min is reached.

NTG is contraindicated in patients who have taken a phosphodiesterase inhibitor for erectile dysfunction within 24 hours. Patients also should not take a phosphodiesterase inhibitor within 24 hours of NTG use. NTG should be used cautiously in patients at risk for severe hypotension, including those with aortic stenosis or right ventricular infarction. NTG should be tapered off slowly because abrupt discontinuation may cause rebound ischemia. Major side effects of NTG include headaches, hypotension, and methemoglobinemia (rare).

NTG is a peripheral and coronary vasodilator. NTG reduces preload via venous dilation, and achieves modest afterload reduction via arterial dilation. These effects result in decreased myocardial oxygen demand. In addition, NTG induces coronary vasodilation, thereby increasing oxygen delivery.

An overview of small, uncontrolled studies has suggested a mortality benefit; however, both the Fourth International Study of Infarct Survival (ISIS-4) and Gruppo Italiano Sperimentazione Streptochinasi Infarto Miocardico - 3 (GISSI-3) studies have failed to confirm these findings.

Morphine Sulfate

Morphine sulfate (MS) should be given to patients who do not respond to anti-ischemic therapy with NTG and beta-blockers or patients who are severely agitated or have pulmonary congestion (ACC/AHA Class I indication). MS is given as an initial dose of 1 to 5 mg intravenously. This may be repeated every 10 minutes to control symptoms, if needed.

The major adverse reactions to MS are hypotension, respiratory depression, nausea, and vomiting. These effects can be reversed with intravenous naloxone 0.4 to 2 mg.

In addition to its analgesic properties, MS also causes venodilation and reduces heart rate. There are no randomized controlled trials examining the benefit of MS in UA/NSTEMI.

Beta-Blockers

Beta-blockers should be used in all patients without contraindications who present with UA/NSTEMI, and should be initially administered intravenously in high-risk patients, and patients with ongoing ischemic symptoms (ACC/AHA Class I indication). The target heart rate for beta-blocker therapy is 50 to 60 bpm. The dosages of commonly used beta-blockers are described in the following text:

- Metoprolol
  - 5 mg IV over 2 min, repeated every 5 min for a total of 15 mg, as tolerated

- ○ 15 min after the last IV dose, initiate 25–50 mg orally every 6 hr for 48 hr
- ○ Maintenance dosing of 50–200 mg orally twice a day
- Atenolol
  - ○ 5 mg IV, repeated in 5 min, as tolerated
  - ○ 1–2 hr after the last IV dose, initiate 50–100 mg orally per day
  - ○ Maintenance dosing of 50–200 mg orally daily
- Propanolol
  - ○ 0.5–1 mg IV
  - ○ 1–2 hr after the initial IV dose, initiate 40–80 mg orally every 6–8 hr
  - ○ Maintenance dosing of 20–80 mg orally twice a day
- Esmolol
  - ○ Continuous intravenous infusion at 0.1 mg/kg/min
  - ○ Increase by 0.05 mg/kg/min every 10–15 min as tolerated, to a maximum dose of 0.3 mg/kg/min

Relative contraindication to the acute use of beta-blockers include severe first-degree or any severity of second- or third-degree atrioventricular block without a pacemaker, history of reactive airways disease, left ventricular dysfunction with congestive heart failure, severe hypotension, shock with systolic blood pressure less than 100 mmHg, or bradycardia.

Beta-blockers decrease heart rate and cardiac contractility via the beta-1-adrenergic receptor, thereby decreasing myocardial oxygen demand. The reduction in heart rate also increases the duration of diastole, which results in increased coronary perfusion.

Beta-blockers decrease mortality and morbidity in patients with acute MI, angina, and heart failure.

Calcium channel blockers

Nondihydropyridine calcium channel blockers (CCB), such as diltiazem and verapamil, may be used in patients with ongoing ischemia when beta-blockers are contraindicated (ACC/AHA Class I indication), or when beta-blockers and NTG have been maximized (ACC/AHA Class IIa indication). Diltiazem 30 to 80 mg orally four times daily (120–320 mg daily for the slow-release formulation) or verapamil 80 to 160 mg orally three times a day (120–480 mg daily for the slow-release formulation) may be used.

The major side effects of CCBs include hypotension, bradycardia, AV nodal blockade, and exacerbation of heart failure. Therefore, diltiazem and verapamil should be avoided in patients with congestive heart failure or pulmonary edema. In patients with adequate beta-blockade, amlodipine and nifedipine may be used (ACC/AHA Class IIB indication).

Calcium channel blockers inhibit myocardial and smooth muscle contraction, leading to decreased myocardial oxygen demand through decreased cardiac contractility and after-load reduction. In addition, coronary perfusion may also improve due to the vasodilatory effects of CCBs.

Nondihydropyridine CCBs are not harmful in patients with ACS, and some data show a trend toward a mortality benefit. One study showed that diltiazem reduced the rate of death, MI, ischemia at 6 months. On the other hand, dihydropyridine CCBs, such as amlodipine and nifedipine, have been shown to increase the risk of MI or recurrent ischemia when not used in conjunction with a beta-blocker. In summary, nondihydropyridine CCBs are not necessarily deleterious when used with a beta-blocker, this combination may have a beneficial effect in patients with ACS.

ACE inhibitors

ACE-I should be used in patients with diabetes mellitus or left ventricular systolic dysfunction who have persistent hypertension after therapy with NTG and a beta-blocker (ACC/AHA Class I indication).

Anti-Platelet Therapy

Aspirin, clopidogrel, and GP IIb/IIIa inhibitors are the main agents used for anti-platelet therapy.

Aspirin

Aspirin should be initiated as early as possible and continued indefinitely (ACC/AHA Class I indication). The initial dose of 162 to 325 mg of non-enteric-coated aspirin should be chewed for rapid absorption. Maintenance dosing with enteric-coated aspirin 81 to 162 mg daily should be used thereafter.

The major side effects of aspirin are gastro-intestinal ulcers and bleeding, aspirin-induced asthma, and bleeding. Therefore, contraindications and cautions for aspirin use include active bleeding, history of severe gastrointestinal bleeding, and asthma.

Aspirin inhibits cyclooxygenase 1, preventing the formation of thromboxane A2 and diminishing platelet aggregation.

Aspirin has been shown to decrease mortality rates in patients with acute myocardial infarction.

Clopidogrel

Clopidogrel should be administered:

- To patients who are unable to take aspirin (ACC/AHA Class I indication)
- In addition to aspirin for patients in whom a conservative noninvasive strategy is planned (ACC/AHA Class I indication). Clopidogrel should be continued for a minimum of 1 month and up to 9 months
- To patients in whom a percutaneous coronary intervention (PCI) is planned. Clopidogrel should be continued

for a minimum of 1 month and up to 9 months
- Clopidogrel should not be given 5–7 days before a CABG since this increases the risk of major bleeding.

From a practical standpoint, clopidogrel should be used as follows:

- Patients who will not undergo cardiac catheterization should receive clopidogrel 300 mg orally as a loading dose, followed by 75 mg orally daily
- Patients who will undergo an early invasive strategy within 24–36 hr should not initially receive clopidogrel. Based on cardiac catheterization results:
  - Clopidogrel should be withheld if CABG will be performed
  - Clopidogrel may then be initiated using either the 300 or 600 mg loading dose, followed by 75 mg orally daily if CABG will not be performed
- Patients who are unlikely to have a cardiac catheterization performed within the first 24–36 hr should receive clopidogrel 300 mg orally as a loading dose, followed by 75 mg orally daily

The major side effects of clopidogrel are rash, diarrhea, bleeding, and rare cases of thrombotic thrombocytopenic purpura and neutropenia. Clopidogrel is contraindicated in patients with active bleeding.

The Clopidogrel versus Aspirin in Patients at Risk of Ischaemic Events (CAPRIE) trial has shown that clopidogrel is as effective as aspirin for the secondary prevention of myocardial infarction. The Clopidogrel in Unstable Angina to Prevent Recurrent Events (CURE) trial demonstrated that aspirin and clopidogrel co-administration is superior to aspirin alone for reducing the risk of cardiovascular death, myocardial infarction, and stroke in patients with unstable angina. The PCI-CURE trial (a subset of the CURE trial) demonstrated that aspirin and clopidogrel is superior to aspirin alone in patients undergoing PCI. Patients receiving combination therapy had a lower risk of cardio-vascular death, MI and need for urgent revas-cularization when compared to patients who received aspirin alone.

GP IIb/IIIa Inhibitors

Abciximab, eptifibatide, and tirofiban are members of a class of anti-platelet agents known as GP IIb/IIIa inhibitors. Eptifibatide and tirofiban are more commonly used than abciximab. GP IIb/IIIa inhibitors should be used:

- Along with aspirin and heparin in patients who will undergo cardiac catheterization and revascularization (ACC/AHA Class I indication)
- Along with aspirin, heparin, and clopidogrel in patients who will undergo cardiac cathe-terization and revascularization (ACC/AHA Class IIa indication)
- Along with aspirin and heparin in patients with ongoing ischemia, increased cardiac injury markers, or other high-risk features (see TIMI risk score and ACC/AHA risk stratification already discussed) who will not undergo invasive intervention (ACC/AHA Class IIa indication). This recom-mendation applies to eptifibatide and tirofiban only

GP IIb/IIIa inhibitors should be used in conjunction with heparin. The dosing for GP IIb/IIIa inhibitors follows:

- Eptifibatide:
  - For UA/NSTEMI:
    - 180 μg/kg (maximum dose 22.6 mg) bolus given IV over 1–2 min, then 2 μg/

kg/min (maximum rate 15 mg/hr) con-
tinuous IV infusion
- May be given for up to 72 hr
○ For PCI:
  - 180 μg/kg (maximum dose 22.6 mg)
    bolus given IV over 1–2 min, immedi-
    ately prior to PCI, then 2 μg/kg/min
    (maximum rate 15 mg/hr)
    continuous IV infusion for up to
    72 hr
  - Second bolus of 180 μg/kg (maximum
    dose 22.6 mg) IV given 10 min after the
    first bolus
- Tirofiban:
  ○ 0.4 μg/kg/min continuous intravenous
    infusion for 30 min, then 0.1 μg/kg/min
  ○ May continue through and up to 24 hr
    after angiography and PCI
- Abciximab:
  ○ Unstable angina with anticipated PCI
    within 24 hr:
    - 0.25 mg/kg IV bolus, then 10 μg/min
      continuous IV infusion for up to 24 hr,
      ending 1 hr after PCI
- Prevention of restenosis:
  ○ 0.25 mg/kg IV bolus 10–60 min prior to
    procedure, then 0.125 μg/kg/min (up to
    10 μg/min maximum rate) continuous IV
    infusion for 12 hr

The major side effects of GP IIb/IIIa inhibitors are bleeding, thrombocytopenia, nausea,
and hypotension. Use of GP IIb/IIIa inhibitors
are contraindicated in patients with active
bleeding, a bleeding diathesis within the preceding 30 days, history of stroke within the
preceding 30 days, major surgery within
the previous 6 weeks, and hypertension with
systolic blood pressure greater than 200 mmHg
or diastolic blood pressure greater than
110 mmHg. GP IIb/IIIa inhibitors should not be

used in patients allergic to any component of the product.

GP IIb/IIIa receptor inhibitors prevent the GP IIb/IIIa receptor (located on platelet surfaces) from binding fibrinogen, resulting in decreased platelet aggregation.

A number of studies have evaluated the efficacy of G IIb/IIIa inhibitors in ACS. Both the Platelet Receptor Inhibition in Ischemic Syndrome Management (PRISM) and Platelet Receptor Inhibition in Ischemic Syndrome Management in Patients Limited by Unstable Signs and Syndromes (PRISM-PLUS) studies demonstrated a short-term mortality reduction with tirofiban. This benefit was seen mainly in higher risk patients with abnormal cardiac markers and ST-segment or T-wave changes. The Platelet Glycoprotein IIb/IIIa in Unstable Angina: Receptor Suppression Using Integrilin Therapy (PURSUIT) trial evaluated the use of eptifibatide in patients with chest pain and CK–MB elevation with ST-segment or T-wave changes. Use of eptifibatide resulted in a reduction in death or non-fatal MI at 6 months.

Anticoagulants

Heparin

Either IV unfractionated heparin (UFH) or subcutaneous low molecular weight heparin (LMWH) should be given in addition to antiplatelet therapy with aspirin and/or clopidogrel (ACC/AHA Class I indication). The dosages for LMWH and UFH are given as follows:

- Enoxaparin:
  - 1 mg/kg subcutaneously every 12 hr
  - An initial 30 mg IV bolus may be given
- Dalteparin:
  - 120 IU/kg subcutaneously every 12 hr

- ○ Maximum dose is 10,000 IU every 12 hr
- Unfractionated heparin:
  - ○ 60–70 U/kg (maximum 5000 U) IV bolus
  - ○ Follow with 12–15 U/kg/hr (maximum 1000 U/hr), titrated to aPTT 1.5 to 2 times control

For patients planning to undergo cardiac catheterization and/or PCI, LMWH may be used during initial stabilization and then switched to UFH the morning of the procedure.

The major side effects of heparin are bleeding and development of heparin-induced thrombocytopenia (HIT). Heparin is contraindicated in patients with active bleeding, a history of HIT, or hypersensitivity to any of its components.

UFH accelerates the action of antithrombin, causing inactivation of procoagulant factors IIa, IXa, and Xa. LMWH agents exert their effects primarily via inhibition of factor Xa.

UFH reduces the risk of MI and recurrent refractory angina. UFH also reduces short-term (but not long-term) mortality. LMWH reduces the short-term (6-day) risk of death, MI, and need for revascularization, with a nonsignificant reduction for risk of death or MI at 40 days.

When LMWH and UFH were compared, two studies—Thrombolysis in MI (TIMI) 11B and Efficacy and Safety of Subcutaneous Enoxaparin in Non-Q Wave Coronary Events (ESSENCE)—found that LMWH had a lower risk of death, MI, and recurrent ischemia than UFH. However, FRIC and FRAXIS found a nonsignificant lower risk of death, MI, and recurrent ischemia with UFH.

Direct Thrombin Inhibitors

Lepirudin and hirudin may be used instead of heparin for patients with a history of HIT.

Thrombolytic Agents

Thrombolytic agents do not improve clinical outcomes in patients with UA/NSTEMI and should not be used.

Conservative Medical Management vs Early Invasive Strategy

An ACC/AHA Class I indication for early coronary angiography exists for patients with UA/NSTEMI and:

- Cardiogenic shock or hemodynamic instability
- Left ventricular dysfunction resulting in heart failure (ejection fraction < 40%), S_3 gallop, pulmonary edema, or mitral regurgitation
- Recurrent angina or ischemia despite maximal medical therapy
- Elevated cardiac injury markers
- New ST-segment depression
- Sustained ventricular tachycardia
- PCI within 6 months or history of CABG
- Noninvasive stress testing that reveals high-risk features

In general, an early invasive strategy refers to coronary angiography and revascularization within 24 hours of presentation. Multiple studies (TACTICS-TIMI, RITA-3, FRISC II, etc.) have shown that an early invasive strategy benefits patients at high-risk for adverse outcomes. Therefore, an early invasive strategy should be pursued in patients with a TIMI risk score greater than 3, or with an ACC/AHA category of intermediate or high risk (see preceding text).

Patients at low risk of adverse outcomes (TIMI risk score 0–2 or ACC/AHA category of low risk) are less likely to benefit from an invasive strategy. These patients may be managed using early invasive strategy or conservative medical therapy.

REFERENCES

Guidelines

1. Braunwald E, Antman EM, Beasley JW, et al. ACC/AHA 2002 guideline update for the management of patients with unstable angina and non-ST-segment elevation myocardial infarction: A report of the American College of Cardiology/American Heart Association Task Force on Practice Guidelines (Committee on the Management of Patients with Unstable Angina). 2002. Available at: http://www.acc.org/clinical/guidelines/unstable/unstable.pdf.
2. Braunwald E, Antman EM, Beasley JW, et al. ACC/AHA 2002 guideline update for the management of patients with unstable angina and non-ST-segment elevation myocardial infarction: Summary article: A report of the American College of Cardiology/American Heart Association Task Force on Practice Guidelines (Committee on the Management of Patients with Unstable Angina). *J Am Coll Cardiol*. 2002;40:1366–1374.
3. Harrington RA, Becker RC, Ezekowitz M, et al. Antithrombotic therapy for coronary artery disease: The Seventh ACCP Conference on Antithrombotic and Thrombolytic Therapy. *Chest* 2004;126:513S–548S.

Review Articles

1. Yeghiazarians Y, Braunstein JB, Askari A, et al. Unstable angina pectoris. *N Engl J Med*. 2000;342:101–114.

Risk Score

1. Antman EM, Cohen M, Bernink PJ, et al. The TIMI risk score for unstable angina/non-ST elevation MI: A method for prognostication and therapeutic decision making. *JAMA* 2000;284:835–842.

Anti-Ischemic Agents

1. Karlberg KE, Saldeen T, Wallin R, et al. Intravenous nitroglycerin reduces ischaemia in unstable angina pectoris: A double-blind placebo-controlled study. *J Int Med.* 1998;243:25–31.
2. Early treatment of unstable angina in the coronary care unit: A randomised, double blind, placebo controlled comparison of recurrent ischaemia in patients treated with nifedipine or metoprolol or both. Report of The Holland Interuniversity Nifedipine/Metoprolol Trial (HINT) Research Group. *Br Heart J.* 1986;56:400–413.
3. Brunner M, Faber TS, Greve B, et al. Usefulness of carvedilol in unstable angina pectoris. *Am J Cardiol.* 2000;85:1173–1178.

Anti-Platelet Agents

1. Collaborative meta-analysis of randomised trials of antiplatelet therapy for prevention of death, myocardial infarction, and stroke in high risk patients. *BMJ* 2002;324:71–86.
2. Fox KA, Mehta SR, Peters R, et al. Benefits and risks of the combination of clopidogrel and aspirin in patients undergoing surgical revascularization for non-ST-elevation acute coronary syndrome: The Clopidogrel in Unstable angina to prevent Recurrent ischemic Events (CURE) Trial. *Circulation* 2004;110:1202–1208.
3. Mehta SR, Yusuf S, Peters RJG, et al, for the Clopidogrel in Unstable angina to prevent Recurrent Events trial (CURE)

Investigators. Effects of pretreatment with clopidogrel and aspirin followed by long-term therapy in patients undergoing percutaneous coronary intervention: The PCI-CURE study. *Lancet* 2001;358:527–533.

4. Cannon CP. Effectiveness of clopidogrel versus aspirin in preventing acute myocardial infarction in patients with symptomatic atherothrombosis (CAPRIE trial). *Am J Cardiol.* 2002;90:760–762.

5. Inhibition of the platelet glycoprotein IIb/IIIa receptor with tirofiban in unstable angina and non-Q-wave myocardial infarction Platelet Receptor Inhibition in Ischemic Syndrome Management in Patients Limited by Unstable Signs and Symptoms (PRISM-PLUS) Study Investigators. *N Engl J Med.* 1998;338:1488–1497.

6. A comparison of aspirin plus tirofiban with aspirin plus heparin for unstable angina. Platelet Receptor Inhibition in Ischemic Syndrome Management (PRISM) Study Investigators. *N Engl J Med.* 1998;338:1498–1505.

7. Inhibition of platelet glycoprotein IIb/IIIa with eptifibatide in patients with acute coronary syndromes. The PURSUIT Trial Investigators. Platelet Glycoprotein IIb/IIIa in Unstable Angina: Receptor Suppression Using Integrilin Therapy. *N Engl J Med.* 1998;339:436–443.

8. Kleiman NS, Lincoff AM, Flaker GC, et al. Early percutaneous coronary intervention, platelet inhibition with eptifibatide, and clinical outcomes in patients with acute coronary syndromes. *Circulation* 2000;101:751–757.

Heparin

1. Oler A, Whooley MA, Oler J, et al. Adding heparin to aspirin reduces the incidence of myocardial infarction and death in patients with unstable angina. *JAMA* 1996;276:811–815.

2. Goodman SG, Cohen M, Bigonzi F, et al. Randomized trial of low molecular weight heparin (enoxaparin) versus unfractionated heparin for unstable coronary artery disease: One-year results of the ESSENCE Study. Efficacy and Safety of Subcutaneous Enoxaparin in Non-Q Wave Coronary Events. *J Am Coll Cardiol.* 2000; 36:693–698.

3. Antman EM, McCabe CH, Gurfinkel EP, et al. Enoxaparin prevents death and cardiac ischemic events in unstable angina/non-Q-wave myocardial infarction: Results of the Thrombolysis In Myocardial Infarction (TIMI) 11B trial. *Circulation* 1999;100:1593–1601.

4. Comparison of two treatment durations (6 days and 14 days) of a low molecular weight heparin with a 6-day treatment of unfractionated heparin in the initial management of unstable angina or non-Q wave myocardial infarction: FRAX.I.S. (FRAxiparine in Ischaemic Syndrome). *Eur Heart J.* 1999;20:1553–1562.

5. Klein W, Buchwald A, Hillis SE, et al, for the FRIC Investigators. Comparison of low-molecular-weight heparin with unfractionated heparin acutely and with placebo for 6 weeks in the management of unstable coronary artery disease. Fragmin in Unstable Coronary Artery Disease Study (FRIC). *Circulation* 1997;96:61–68.

Early Invasive Strategy

1. Cannon CP, Weintraub WS, Demopoulos LA, et al. Comparison of early invasive and conservative strategies in patients with unstable coronary syndromes treated with the glycoprotein IIb/IIIa inhibitor tirofiban. *N Engl J Med.* 2001;344:1879–1887.

2. Fox K, Poole-Wilson P, Henderson R, et al. Interventional versus conservative treatment for patients with unstable angina or

non-ST-elevation myocardial infarction:
The British Heart Foundation RITA 3
randomised trial. *Lancet* 2002;360:743–751.
3. Mehta SR, Cannon CP, Fox KA,
et al. Routine vs selective invasive strategies
in patients with acute coronary syndromes:
A collaborative meta-analysis of randomized
trials. *JAMA* 2005;293:2908–2917.

Endocrinology

C H A P T E R 4

Adrenal Insufficiency

KEY POINTS

1. The most common cause of adrenal insufficiency (AI) is exogenous glucocorticoid use in patients taking more than the equivalent of prednisone 5 mg orally daily for longer than 3 weeks.

2. A morning cortisol level greater than 18 to 20 µg/dL essentially rules out AI. Levels less than 3 µg/dL are highly suggestive of AI. Patients with a morning cortisol level less than 18 to 20 µg/dL should undergo an ACTH stimulation test.

3. Cortisol levels less than 18 to 20 µg/dL on ACTH stimulation testing confirm the diagnosis of AI. Primary AI is associated with a high baseline ACTH level. Secondary AI is associated with a low baseline ACTH level.

4. Maintenance therapy for AI is the equivalent of hydrocortisone 15 to 20 mg orally in the morning and 5 to 10 mg orally at night.

5. The maintenance dose should be doubled or tripled for mild illness. Moderate illness requires hydrocortisone 50 mg twice a day. Severe illness requires hydrocortisone 100 mg every 8 hours.

6. Functional and relative adrenal insufficiency during critical illness should be suspected in patients with continuing hypotension despite adequate volume repletion. Treatment is hydrocortisone 50 mg intravenously given every 8 hours.

Box 4-1. Causes of Primary Adrenal Insufficiency

- Idiopathic/Autoimmune: ~80%
- Tuberculosis: Slightly less than 20%
- Other: ~1%
  - Vascular
    - Hemorrhage: sepsis, anticoagulation, coagulopathy, trauma, surgery, pregnancy, neonate
    - Infarction: thrombosis, embolism, arteritis
  - Fungal infection
    - Histoplasmosis
    - Blastomycosis
    - Coccidioidomycosis
    - Cryptococcosis
  - HIV
  - Infiltrative diseases
    - Metastases
    - Lymphoma
    - Amyloidosis
    - Sarcoidosis
    - Hemochromatosis
  - Iatrogenic
    - Radiation
    - Surgery (bilateral adrenalectomy)
    - Drugs
      - Mitotane
      - Enzyme inhibitors (ketoconazole, etomidate, metyrapone, trilostane, aminoglutethimide
  - Congenital
    - Adrenal hypoplasia
    - Familial glucocorticoid deficiency
    - Adrenal leukodystrophy

DEFINITION AND EPIDEMIOLOGY

Primary adrenal insufficiency occurs when the adrenal glands fail to produce enough corticosteroids to meet the body's needs. Approximately

90% of adrenal mass must be lost before this condition occurs.

Primary adrenal insufficiency is a rare condition, with a prevalence of 40 to 60 cases per million. Historically, tuberculosis accounted for the majority of cases. Currently, autoimmune adrenalitis accounts for approximately 80% of cases, tuberculosis accounts for less than 20%; the remaining 1% of cases are due to other miscellaneous causes (Box 4-1).

Secondary adrenal insufficiency is caused by failure of the pituitary gland to produce enough ACTH to maintain cortisol production by the adrenal glands. Exogenous administration of glucocorticoids is the most common cause of secondary adrenal insufficiency. Non-iatrogenic causes, such as pituitary apoplexy, infarction, hemorrhage, or tumors, are uncommon.

ETIOLOGY

We will briefly discuss a few of the more common causes of primary adrenal insufficiency (see Box 4-1).

Autoimmune Adrenalitis

Evidence of autoimmune attack against all three zones of the adrenal cortex is present. Antibodies to 17 alpha hydroxylase and 21 hydroxylase are present in 65% of patients, although the role of these auto-antibodies is unclear. There is an association between autoimmune adrenalitis and other autoimmune diseases, which will be discussed.

Polyglandular Autoimmune Syndrome Type I (PAS I)

The classic triad of PAS I is hypoparathyroidism, chronic mucocutaneous candidiasis, and adrenal insufficiency. PAS I usually presents by age 5, with clinical manifestations complete by age 15.

Box 4-2. Medications That Increase Glucocorticoid Metabolism

Patients treated with these medications may need higher replacement doses of glucocorticoids

- Phenytoin
- Rifampin
- Mitotane
- Barbiturates
- Aminoglutethimide

Typically, hypoparathyroidism or candidiasis occurs first, with adrenal insufficiency presenting in the early teens.

In some patients, PAS I is also associated with gonadal failure, autoimmune thyroiditis, and type 1 diabetes mellitus. There is no HLA association. PAS I is commonly associated with other autoimmune diseases, such as pernicious anemia, vitiligo, and alopecia. Siblings of the proband should be screened for PAS I at regular screenings.

Polyglandular Autoimmune Syndrome Type II (PAS II)

PAS II is the more common form of polyglandular autoimmune syndrome, and occurs mainly in adults between the third and fifth decades of life. There is at least a 2:1 female predominance. The classic triad is adrenal insufficiency, autoimmune thyroid disease, and type 1 diabetes mellitus.

PAS II is not usually associated with other auto-immune diseases except vitiligo.

Other Causes

Although clinical adrenal insufficiency is rare, the adrenals are involved in up to 85% of cases of terminal tuberculosis. In patients with HIV, aty-

Box 4-3. Corticosteroid Replacement Dosing

Maintenance Therapy

Otherwise healthy patients, or patients with a non-febrile, minor illness

- Prednisone 5 mg (2.5–7.5 mg) orally at bedtime
- Dexamethasone 0.5 mg (0.25–0.75 mg) orally at bedtime
- Hydrocortisone 15–20 mg orally in the morning, and 5–10 mg orally at night
- Assess replacement adequacy clinically, and with morning ACTH levels

Mineralocorticoid Therapy

For patients with primary adrenal insufficiency

- Fludrocortisone 0.1 mg (0.05–0.2 mg) orally daily
- Lower doses are usually required when using hydrocortisone
- Higher doses are usually required when using prednisone or dexamethasone
- Assess adequacy of replacement using orthostatic vital signs, serum sodium and potassium levels, and plasma renin activity

Minor Illness or Procedure

Mild febrile illness, or procedures performed under local anesthesia, dental procedures, or most radiologic studies

- Outpatient management: use two or three times maintenance dose during illness, then return to maintenance dose. If illness does not resolve in 3 days, contact physician
- Inpatient management: use two or three times maintenance dose until 24 hr after resolution of illness, then resume maintenance dose

Continued

Box 4-3. Corticosteroid Replacement Dosing—cont'd

- Consider IV glucocorticoids (methylprednisolone) in patients who cannot tolerate oral medications
- For minor procedures, take maintenance dose only

Moderate Illness

- Hydrocortisone 50 mg orally or IV twice a day (or equivalent)
- Taper rapidly over 1–2 days to maintenance dose after patient recovers

Severe Illness

- Hydrocortisone 100 mg IV every 8 hr
- Adjust dose according to patient's condition
- Taper rapidly over 1–2 days to maintenance dose after patient recovers

Moderately Stressful Procedures

Including endoscopy, barium enema, arteriography

- Hydrocortisone 100 mg IV before the procedure

Major Surgery

- Hydrocortisone 100 mg IV just before induction of anesthesia
- Continue hydrocortisone 100 mg IV every 8 hr for the first 24 hr
- If no complications occur, taper by 50% per day to maintenance dosage

Precautions

- Patients should wear a medic-alert bracelet
- Patients should carry syringes with 4 mg of dexamethasone in 1 mL of saline

From Stewart PM. In: Williams RH, Larsen PR, and Kronenberg HM, et al, editors. *Williams' Textbook of Endocrinology*, 10th ed., Philadelphia. Elsevier. Copyright © 2003 Elsevier. Reproduced with permission, 2005.

pical mycobacteria, such as *mycobacterium avium-intracellulare*, may cause adrenal insufficiency. Cytomegalovirus infection is another cause of adrenal insufficiency in patients with HIV.

Disseminated histoplasmosis results in adrenal insufficiency in up to 50% of cases. Other fungal

Table 4-1. Manifestations of Primary Adrenal Insufficiency

Symptoms	Frequency (%)
Weakness, tiredness, fatigue	100
Anorexia	100
Gastrointestinal symptoms	92
Nausea	86
Vomiting	75
Constipation	33
Abdominal pain	31
Diarrhea	16
Salt craving	16
Postural dizziness	12
Muscle or joint pains	6–13
Signs	**Frequency (%)**
Weight loss	100
Hyperpigmentation	94
Hypotension (<110 mm Hg systolic)	88–94
Vitiligo	10–20
Auricular calcification	5
Laboratory Finding	**Frequency (%)**
Electrolyte disturbances	92
Hyponatremia	88
Hyperkalemia	64
Hypercalcemia	6
Azotemia	55
Anemia	40
Eosinophilia	17

From Stewart PM. In: Williams RH, Larsen PR, and Kronenberg HM, et al, editors. *Williams' Textbook of Endocrinology*, 10th ed., Philadelphia. Elsevier. Copyright © 2003 Elsevier. Reproduced with permission, 2005.

infections, such as paracoccidioidomycosis, blastomycosis, coccidioidomycosis, and cryptococcus cause adrenal insufficiency much less frequently.

Metastatic tumors are a rare cause of adrenal insufficiency, because 90% of total adrenal mass must be destroyed before symptoms develop.

Special Cases

Exogenous glucocorticoid administration is the most common cause of adrenal insufficiency. The administration of greater than 5 mg of prednisone (or equivalent) for longer than three weeks may result in suppression of the hypothalamic–pituitary–adrenal axis, and result in adrenal insufficiency during times of stress or medication non-compliance. These patients should be treated with supplemental glucocorticoids during stressful periods (Box 4-3).

Functional and relative adrenal insufficiency may occur in patients with critical illness, such as septic shock, and treatment with glucocorticoids may improve outcomes.

CLINICAL FEATURES

Adrenal Crisis

Adrenal crisis may be the presentation of a previously undiagnosed case of adrenal insufficiency, or may occur in a patient with known adrenal insufficiency who is unable to increase their corticosteroid dosage (due to nausea, vomiting, or unexpected trauma) (see Box 4-3). Adrenal crisis is primarily a manifestation of primary adrenal insufficiency, because hypotension is caused mainly by mineralocorticoid deficiency exacerbated by low glucocorticoid levels. In contrast, the renin-angiotensin-aldosterone system is preserved in secondary or tertiary AI.

In addition to the typical signs and symptoms of primary adrenal insufficiency (Table 4-1),

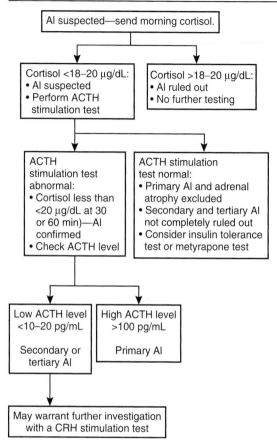

FIGURE 4–1. Algorithm for diagnosis of adrenal insufficiency (AI).

patients with adrenal crisis usually have abdominal pain, nausea and vomiting, fever, and hypoglycemia.

Chronic Primary Adrenal Insufficiency

Generalized complaints of fatigue, malaise, and anorexia occur in virtually all patients. Orthostatic hypotension, rather than shock, characterizes chronic adrenal insufficiency. Gastrointestinal symptoms are common, with 92% of patients reporting abdominal pain, nausea, vomiting, or changes in bowel habits.

Hyperpigmentation may be found in patients with primary adrenal insufficiency, due to increased melanocyte stimulating hormone levels, but is absent in secondary adrenal insufficiency. In patients with darker skin, such as African Americans, inspection of the buccal mucosa or palmar folds may be helpful. Hyperpigmentation may also manifest as darker hair or nail color.

Hyponatremia and hyperkalemia are noted in 88% and 64% of patients with primary AI, respectively. Hypoglycemia, or decreased insulin requirements in patients with type 1 diabetes, may occur.

In patients with polyglandular autoimmune syndromes, signs and symptoms of associated conditions may be evident.

The major findings in primary adrenal insufficiency are described in Table 4-1.

DIAGNOSIS (Fig. 4-1)

Laboratory Testing

Morning Cortisol Level

The first diagnostic step is to confirm that the cortisol level is abnormally low by checking a morning cortisol level around 8:00 AM (Fig. 4-1). A morning cortisol level greater than 18 to 20 µg/dL essentially rules out adrenal insufficiency, and further testing is not routinely necessary. Conversely, levels less than 3 µg/dL are virtually diagnostic of adrenal insufficiency. For patients with a basal morning cortisol level less than 18 to 20 µg/dL, further testing with an ACTH stimulation test is necessary.

ACTH Stimulation Test

The steps to performing the ACTH stimulation test are as follows:

- Draw a baseline serum ACTH and cortisol level.
- Administer 250 µg of cosyntropin (synthetic ACTH) intravenously.
- Measure serum cortisol and aldosterone level at 30 and 60 minutes after administration of cosyntropin.

Normal cortisol levels

If the cortisol level at 30 or 60 minutes is greater than 18 to 20 µg/dL, primary adrenal insufficiency has been ruled out, as have the majority of cases of secondary adrenal insufficiency. Long-standing secondary adrenal insufficiency results in adrenal atrophy, which would blunt the cortisol response of cosyntropin administration. However, chronic partial ACTH deficiency and new-onset (<1 month) secondary adrenal insufficiency may be missed. In chronic partial ACTH deficiency, there may be enough ACTH produced to preserve some adrenal function. In new-onset secondary adrenal insufficiency, the adrenals may not have atrophied yet. These uncommon cases may be assessed with an insulin tolerance test or a metyrapone test (metyrapone is available only by special order from Novartis). Contraindications for insulin tolerance testing include a history of seizures or coronary artery disease.

Table 4-2. Equivalent Glucocorticoid Doses	
Drug	**Dose (mg)**
Prednisone	1
Prednisolone	1
Hydrocortisone	4
Methylprednisolone	0.8
Dexamethasone	0.15

Low cortisol levels

Cortisol levels below 18 to 20 µg/dL at 30 or 60 minutes confirms the diagnosis of adrenal insufficiency. If the baseline ACTH level is high (100 pg/mL), the patient has primary adrenal insufficiency, whereas if the baseline ACTH level is low (10–20 pg/mL), the diagnosis is either secondary or tertiary adrenal insufficiency. To distinguish between the latter two diagnoses, a CRH stimulation test may be considered. However, a CRH stimulation test is almost never necessary in clinical practice, as there is little practical importance in distinguishing secondary from tertiary adrenal insufficiency.

MANAGEMENT

Chronic Primary Adrenal Insufficiency

Maintenance Therapy

Maintenance therapy of hydrocortisone, 15 to 20 mg in the morning and 5 to 10 mg at night or equivalent (see Table 4-2 for equivalent dosages of glucocorticoids), should be administered. The optimal dose should be individualized for each patient by symptomatic assessment and measurement of morning ACTH levels. Some clinicians prefer the use of longer-acting glucocorticoid preparations, such as prednisone 5 mg/day or dexamethasone 0.5 mg/day.

Mineralocorticoid replacement with fludrocortisone 0.1 mg/day (range of 0.05–0.2 mg/day) should also be given. For patients receiving hydrocortisone, lower doses may be required, because hydrocortisone has some intrinsic mineralocorticoid activity.

Minor Illness or Procedure

For minor procedures performed under local anesthesia, dental procedures, and most radiologic studies, only the usual maintenance dose is required.

Patients with mild febrile illness, such as a viral syndrome or gastroenteritis should increase their glucocorticoid dose by two or three times the maintenance dose. If no resolution is noted in 3 days, the patient should contact the physician. Inpatients with a mild febrile illness should be administered glucocorticoid replacement at three times their maintenance dose until 24 hours after symptom resolution. They should then resume

Box 4-4. Treatment of Adrenal Crisis

Emergency Measures

- Establish intravenous access with large-gauge catheters
- Draw blood for electrolytes, glucose, cortisol and ACTH; do not wait for results before initiating therapy
- Infuse 2–3 L of 0.9% (normal) saline, or D_5 normal saline; observe and monitor for signs of fluid overload
- Administer hydrocortisone 100 mg IV every 6 hr
- Give other supportive care as needed

Other Measures After Patient Stabilization

- Continue 0.9% saline infusion at a slower rate for 24–48 hr
- Investigate and treat precipitants of adrenal crisis
- Confirm diagnosis of adrenal insufficiency, if necessary
- If possible, taper steroids to maintenance dose over 1–3 days
- Start fludrocortisone 0.1 mg orally daily for patients with primary AI when saline infusion is discontinued

From Stewart PM. In: Williams RH, Larsen PR, and Kronenberg HM, et al, editors. *Williams' Textbook of Endocrinology*, 10th ed., Philadelphia. Elsevier. Copyright © 2003 Elsevier. Reproduced with permission, 2005.

their usual maintenance dose. Intravenous administration of glucocorticoids should be administered to patients who cannot take oral medications.

Patients receiving more than 100 mg total daily dose of hydrocortisone usually do not require mineralocorticoid supplementation.

Moderate to Severe Illness

For moderate febrile illness, such as pneumonia, mild diverticulitis, severe gastroenteritis, or other conditions of similar severity, the patient should receive the equivalent of hydrocortisone 50 mg intravenously twice daily. Patients with more severe disease should be given the equivalent of hydrocortisone 100 mg intravenously every 8 hours. In either case, once the patient recovers, the glucocorticoid dose may be rapidly tapered to the maintenance dose over 1 to 2 days.

Other Procedures and Surgery

For endoscopy, angiography, and moderately stressful fluoroscopic procedures such as barium enema, 100 mg of hydrocortisone should be administered before the procedure. For major surgical procedures, including cardiac or major abdominal surgery, 100 mg of hydrocortisone should be given immediately prior to induction of anesthesia. Subsequently, 100 mg of hydrocortisone should be given every 8 hours for the first 24 hours. If no complications occur, this dose may be tapered by 50% per day until the usual maintenance dose is reached.

During labor, 50 mg of hydrocortisone may be given every 6 hours. After delivery, this dose may be tapered rapidly to the maintenance dose.

Adrenal Crisis

The treatment of adrenal crisis is summarized in Box 4-4.

Critical Illness

Functional adrenal insufficiency (inability of the adrenal glands to produce normal levels of corticosteroids during acute illness) or *relative adrenal insufficiency* (lack of ability to control inflammation despite high levels of corticosteroids) may increase mortality during critical illness.

Functional or relative adrenal insufficiency usually manifests as hypotension despite aggressive fluid resuscitation. Hypoglycemia, hyponatremia, or hyperkalemia may also be seen. Maintaining a high index of suspicion is crucial in critically ill patients.

Random Cortisol Level

The first step in testing for functional or relative adrenal insufficiency is obtaining a random serum cortisol level. Levels below 15 µg/dL strongly suggest adrenal insufficiency, and treatment should be considered. Conversely, levels above 34 µg/dL make adrenal insufficiency unlikely, and no further evaluation or therapy is necessary.

Levels between 9 and 34 warrant further investigation with an ACTH stimulation test.

ACTH Stimulation Test

A baseline cortisol level is measured. Then, 250 µg of cosyntropin is administered intravenously, and a cortisol level is measured at 30 and 60 minutes post-injection. An increase in cortisol less than 9 µg/dL from baseline strongly suggests adrenal insufficiency, and treatment should be considered. An increase in cortisol greater than, or equal to, 9 µg/dL makes adrenal insufficiency unlikely, and treatment is not warranted.

Treatment of functional or relative adrenal insufficiency in critical illness is hydrocortisone,

50 mg intravenously every 6 hours. One trial also administered fludrocortisone, 0.05 mg through nasogastric tube daily. Treatment should be continued for 7 days.

REFERENCES

Textbook Chapters

Stewart PM. The adrenal cortex. In: Williams RH, Larsen PR, and Kronenberg HM, et al, editors. *Williams Textbook of Endocrinology*, 10th ed. Philadelphia. Elsevier; 2003: 525–532.

Review Articles

1. Cooper MS, Stewart PM. Corticosteroid insufficiency in acutely ill patients. *N Engl J Med*. 2003;348:727–734.
2. Rivers EP, Gaspari M, Saad GA, et al. Adrenal insufficiency in high-risk surgical ICU patients. *Chest* 2001;119:889–896.
3. Lamberts SWJ, Bruining HA, deJong FH. Corticosteroid therapy in severe illness. *N Engl J Med*. 1997;337:1285–1292.
4. Coursin DB, Wood KE. Corticosteroid supplementation for adrenal insufficiency. *JAMA* 2002;287:236–240.
5. Oelkers W. Adrenal insufficiency. *N Engl J Med*. 1996;335:1206–1212.

Article

Hamrahian AH, Oseni TS, Arafah BM. Measurements of serum free cortisol in critically ill patients. *N Engl J Med*. 2004;350:1629–1638.

CHAPTER 5

Diabetic Ketoacidosis

KEY POINTS

1. Diabetic ketoacidosis (DKA) is characterized by hyperglycemia (blood glucose usually above 300 mg/dL), hyperketonemia, and metabolic acidosis.
2. DKA classically occurs in patients with type 1 diabetes mellitus but can also occasionally develop in patients with type 2 diabetes.
3. The major precipitants of DKA include cessation of insulin (endogenous or exogenous), infection, and stress (such as myocardial infarction or stroke). No precipitating event is identified in up to one fourth of patients.
4. Patients with DKA commonly present with weight loss, polyuria, polydipsia, nausea, vomiting, dehydration, and abdominal pain. Fever is not a feature of DKA itself and suggests underlying infection.
5. On physical examination, patients usually have signs of volume depletion, but may also have Kussmaul respirations (increased ventilation to compensate for the acidemia) and a "fruity breath" odor caused by acetone.
6. Initial laboratory testing should include electrolytes, renal function, serum glucose, complete blood count, liver function tests, urinalysis, ketones (nitroprusside test or beta-hydroxybutyrate), arterial blood gas, serum lactate, creatine phosphokinase, electrocardiogram, chest x-ray, cultures of blood,

urine, and sputum (if applicable), and toxicology screen (if toxic ingestion is suspected).

7. The serum sodium is often factitiously low from dilutional effects caused by the hyperglycemia.

8. The anion gap (representing unmeasured plasma anions) should be elevated in DKA but is also elevated in many other conditions besides DKA.

9. The nitroprusside test may underestimate the degree of ketonemia because it does not detect beta-hydroxybutyrate, which is the predominant circulating ketone body in DKA.

10. DKA is associated with fluid loss (typically 3–6 L), mostly due to osmotic diuresis. Patients with anuric, end-stage renal disease have minimal fluid loss unless there is concurrent vomiting or diarrhea.

11. Normal saline and intravenous regular insulin (5–10 U bolus, then 5–10 U/hr) should be started concurrently. D5 (5% dextrose) should be added to the intravenous fluids when the blood glucose falls below 250 mg/dL.

12. Serum potassium concentrations will decline during treatment as insulin shifts the potassium intracellularly. Potassium 40 mEq/L (less if there is co-existing renal insufficiency) should be added to the intravenous fluids when the serum potassium falls below 4.0 mEq/L.

13. Bicarbonate therapy and phosphate repletion are controversial because these treatments have potential adverse effects and have not been shown to be beneficial in DKA.

14. Transitioning to subcutaneous insulin should only occur when the anion gap

has closed and the patient's appetite has returned. Subcutaneous fast-acting insulin must be administered 30 to 60 minutes before discontinuing the insulin drip; otherwise, DKA may rapidly recur.

EPIDEMIOLOGY

Diabetic ketoacidosis (DKA) classically occurs in patients with type 1 diabetes mellitus but may also occasionally develop in patients with type 2 diabetes. Type 1 diabetes refers to insulin deficiency due to autoimmune destruction of the insulin-producing beta-cells of the pancreas. In the past, type 1 diabetes was called "juvenile" or "insulin-dependent" diabetes. However, these terms are no longer used because this disease can present at any age (patients in their 80s can develop type 1 diabetes), and patients with type 2 diabetes can also be "insulin-dependent." Type 2 diabetes accounts for more than 90% of all cases of diabetes, and it is characterized by relative insulin deficiency and insulin resistance. Type 2 diabetes has been called "non-insulin dependent" or "adult-onset" diabetes, but these terms are also outdated since these patients usually become insulin-dependent as their disease progresses and are presenting at younger ages (even in childhood) because of the increasing obesity epidemic.

The incidence of DKA is 46 to 80 per 10,000 person-years among patients with diabetes, and the estimated mortality rate of DKA is 4% to 10%. Only 20% of DKA episodes occur in patients with new-onset diabetes. Furthermore, 20% of patients with DKA have multiple annual episodes. Therefore, patient education and compliance are crucial for reducing the incidence of DKA.

PATHOGENESIS

The hallmark of DKA is severe insulin deficiency and inappropriate glucagon excess that leads to hyperglycemia and hyperketonemia. Insulin deficiency stimulates hepatic glucose production and causes the release of large amounts of free fatty acids from adipose tissue. The free fatty acids are converted to ketone bodies (acetoacetate and beta-hydroxybutyrate) in the liver, leading to acidosis. Glucagon secretion is inappropriately increased in DKA and directly stimulates ketogenesis as well as gluconeogenesis (glucose production) in the presence of insulin deficiency. The excess glucose production cannot be utilized by muscle or fat (insulin is required for glucose uptake by these tissues), leading to hyperglycemia.

Therefore, the features of DKA are:

1. Hyperglycemia (blood glucose usually > 300 mg/dL)
2. Hyperketonemia
3. Metabolic acidosis (pH < 7.35)

PRECIPITANTS

The major precipitants of DKA (Box 5-1) commonly include cessation of insulin (endogenous or exogenous), infection, and stress (such as myocardial infarction or stroke, but perhaps also emotional stress in certain patients) although no precipitating event is identified in up to one-fourth of patients. Coexisting medical illness is the most common factor and accounts for at least one half of the causes of DKA.

SYMPTOMS

Patients commonly present with polyuria (excessive urination), polydipsia (excessive thirst), nausea, vomiting, and abdominal pain.

Box 5-1. Common Precipitants of Diabetic Ketoacidosis

Infection (even minor or occult, e.g., peri-rectal abscess, furuncle)

  Viral syndrome

  Pneumonia

  Urinary tract infection

Lack of insulin

  Endogenous (newly diagnosed diabetes)

  Exogenous (poor compliance or insufficient insulin)

Stress

  Myocardial infarction

  Stroke

  Surgical abdomen (e.g., mesenteric ischemia, appendicitis)

  Illness

Hypokalemia

No precipitating event identified

Dehydration is typical in DKA because the high urinary glucose concentrations cause diuresis, leading to the usual complaints of polyuria and polydipsia. Weight loss is often a prominent feature in patients with undiagnosed diabetes because their symptoms have typically progressed over several weeks. Fever is not a feature of DKA itself and suggests underlying infection.

SIGNS

On physical examination, patients usually have signs of volume depletion (such as reduced skin turgor, dry mucous membranes, flat jugular veins, tachycardia, hypotension, postural signs), and may also have Kussmaul respirations (increased ventilation compensating for acidemia when the pH < 7.2) or the characteristic "fruity breath" odor caused by high concentrations of acetone. A thorough search for a precipitant, including signs of infection or myocardial infarction (which may present without chest pain in patients with long-standing diabetes), should be undertaken.

LABORATORY DATA

The average laboratory findings in DKA are summarized in Table 5-1.

Initial laboratory testing should include:

1. Electrolytes, renal function, and serum glucose
2. Complete blood count
3. Liver function tests
4. Urinalysis
5. Ketones (nitroprusside test or beta-hydroxybutyrate)
6. Arterial blood gas
7. Serum lactate

The initial search for a precipitant should include:

1. Electrocardiogram and troponins to assess for cardiac ischemia
2. Upright chest x-ray to assess for pneumonia and free air in the peritoneum
3. Blood, urine, and sputum cultures, as indicated
4. Toxicology screen, if toxic ingestion is suspected

A normal chest x-ray may not exclude an underlying pneumonia in dehydrated patients. Therefore, repeat imaging may be necessary after fluid resuscitation if there is suspicion for pneumonia.

Glucose

There is no single blood glucose concentration that can be used to define DKA because some

Table 5-1. Average Laboratory Findings in Diabetic Ketoacidosis

Test	Value	Typical Reference Range
Glucose (mg/dL)	475	54–118
Serum osmolarity (mOsm/kg)	309	278–297
Sodium (mEq/L)	131	135–145
Potassium (mEq/L)	4.8	3.5–5.5
Bicarbonate (mEq/L)	9	23–32
Blood urea nitrogen (mg/dL)	21	9–25
Anion gap (mEq/L)	29	8–12
pH	<7.3	7.35–7.45
Ketonuria	≥3+	0
Beta-hydroxybutyrate (mmol/L)	13.7	0–0.3
Lactate (mmol/L)	4.6	0.5–2.2
Cortisol (µg/dL)	49	3–24
Glucagon (pg/mL)	400–500	25–250

patients with blood glucose concentrations above 400 mg/dL do not have DKA while others have DKA when blood glucose concentrations are less than 350 mg/dL. Lower blood glucose concentrations in the setting of DKA can occur with fasting, alcohol consumption (inhibition of gluconeogenesis), and pregnancy (the fetoplacental unit utilizes glucose in the absence of insulin), but the metabolic acidosis may still be severe.

Sodium

The serum sodium (Na) concentration is often factitiously low from dilutional effects, because hyperglycemia causes osmotic fluid shifts from the intracellular to extracellular compartments. The serum sodium should be corrected for the serum glucose concentration using the following formula:

$$Na\,(corrected) = Measured\,Na + \frac{1.6 \times (glucose\,[mg/dL] - 100\,mg/dL)}{100}$$

Bicarbonate and Anion Gap

The serum bicarbonate attempts to buffer the ketoacids. Therefore, the bicarbonate concentration is usually less than 15 mEq/L and the anion gap (representing unmeasured plasma anions) is typically elevated. The most common method for calculating the anion gap is: Measured Na − (Cl + CO_2) with a normal range of 8 to 12 mEq/L. There are many causes of an elevated anion gap other than DKA, which are summarized by the well-known mnemonic "MUDPILES":

M = methanol
U = uremia
D = DKA
P = paraldehyde
I = iron
L = lactic acidosis
E = ethanol
S = salicylate intoxication

Ketones

Acetoacetate, acetone, and beta-hydroxybutyrate are the three ketone bodies produced in DKA. The nitroprusside test predominantly detects acetoacetate (and, to a much smaller extent, acetone) but does not react with beta-hydroxybutyrate, which is the predominant circulating ketone body in DKA. Therefore, the nitroprusside test may underestimate the true extent of circulating ketone bodies. Direct measurement of beta-hydroxybutyrate circumvents this problem.

There are two other important characteristics of the nitroprusside test: (1) a false positive result can occur in patients receiving captopril, and (2) the test can become more strongly positive as the metabolic derangements of DKA improve and beta-hydroxybutyrate is converted to acetoacetate. However, this is of no consequence provided the anion gap is closing and the patient is continuing to improve clinically.

Other Laboratory Data

Other laboratory abnormalities may include leukocytosis (even in the absence of infection), prerenal azotemia, mild transaminitis, increased creatine phosphokinase concentrations (ranging from mild, asymptomatic elevations to rhabdomyolysis with renal failure), and elevation of serum lipase and amylase concentrations with or without pancreatitis.

TREATMENT (Fig. 5-1)

1. Intravenous Fluids

The typical fluid loss in DKA is 3 to 6 L (Table 5-2) and is mostly the result of osmotic diuresis. Therefore, anuric patients with end-stage renal disease have minimal fluid loss unless there is concurrent vomiting or diarrhea. Initially, normal saline should be used for fluid resuscitation. Half-normal saline should be substituted when the patient's volume deficit has been corrected.

2. Intravenous Insulin

Intravenous insulin should be started concurrently with fluid resuscitation. The recommended

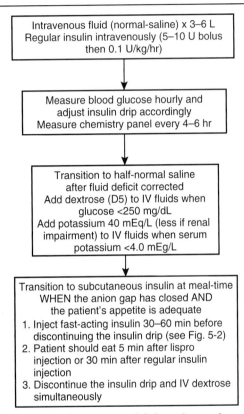

FIGURE 5–1. Initial treatment of diabetic ketoacidosis.

initial intravenous regular insulin regimen is a 0.1 U/kg (5–10 U) bolus followed by an infusion of 0.1 U/kg/hr (5–10 U/hr). Fingerstick blood glucose measurements should be obtained hourly and the insulin drip adjusted accordingly. When the blood glucose is less than 250 mg/dL, we recommend adding 5% dextrose (D5) to the intravenous fluids and continuing the insulin drip. Under no circumstances should the insulin drip be discontinued until the anion gap has closed and rapid-acting subcutaneous insulin has been administered; otherwise, DKA will rapidly worsen.

Table 5-2. Average Water and Electrolyte Deficits in Diabetic Ketoacidosis

Parameter	Deficit
Water (mL/kg)	100
Sodium (mEq/kg)	7–10
Chloride (mEq/kg)	3–5
Potassium (mEq/kg)	3–5
Magnesium (mEq/kg)	1–2
Phosphate (mmol/kg)	1–2

3. Potassium

Initially, the chemistry panel should be obtained at least every 4 to 6 hours. This panel is used to monitor the serum potassium concentration and determine when the anion gap has closed (i.e., when the patient may be ready to transition to subcutaneous insulin). DKA (polyuria, vomiting) typically causes total body potassium depletion (~3–5 mEq/kg). Since insulin is required to move potassium from the extracellular to intracellular compartment, serum potassium levels at presentation are usually normal or high-normal and decline with insulin therapy. Once the serum potassium is less than 4.0 mEq/L, we recommend adding 40 mEq of potassium to each liter of intravenous fluids (smaller amounts of potassium should be added if there is coexisting renal insufficiency).

4. Bicarbonate Therapy

Bicarbonate therapy is controversial. Bicarbonate treatment has not been shown to be beneficial, and the acidosis will correct with insulin and intravenous fluids. Bicarbonate also has theoretical risks of worsening tissue oxygen delivery and increasing lactate production. Bicarbonate therapy is sometimes used transiently if there is severe acidosis (pH < 6.9), hypotension with pH < 7.1, or hyperkalemia with electrocardiographic changes.

5. Phosphate

DKA causes urinary phosphate loss and total body phosphate depletion ($\sim$ 1–2 mEq/kg). As with potassium, serum phosphate levels are typically normal or high at presentation and decline with treatment. However, phosphate repletion is controversial because intravenous phosphate administration may potentially cause severe hypocalcemia and hypomagnesemia and has not been shown to alter the clinical course of DKA. Therefore, we recommend repletion of phosphate stores through dietary phosphate intake only.

TRANSITIONING TO SUBCUTANEOUS INSULIN

Transitioning to subcutaneous insulin should occur only when the anion gap has closed and the patient's appetite has returned, and is easiest to accomplish prior to a meal. The half-life of intravenous insulin is approximately 6 minutes. Therefore, a subcutaneous injection of fast-acting insulin (lispro or regular) is mandated 30 to 60 minutes prior to discontinuation of the insulin drip; otherwise, DKA may rapidly recur. If the patient has a history of diabetes, the home insulin regimen can be restarted, but may need to be modified depending on the circumstances (for example, slight lowering of the insulin dose if there is poor appetite or increase in dose if there is concurrent infection). For a patient with new-onset diabetes, the following algorithm can be used as a starting point to approximate the patient's subcutaneous insulin needs (Fig. 5-2). The patient's daily insulin requirement will

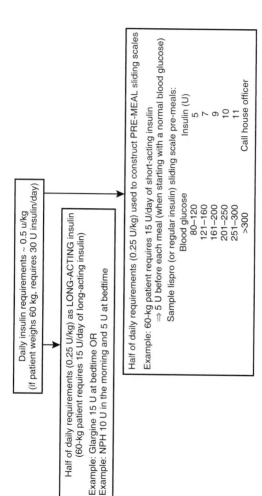

Daily insulin requirements ~ 0.5 u/kg
(if patient weighs 60 kg, requires 30 U insulin/day)

Half of daily requirements (0.25 U/kg) as LONG-ACTING insulin
(60-Kg patient requires 15 U/day of long-acting insulin)

Example: Glargine 15 U at bedtime OR
Example: NPH 10 U in the morning and 5 U at bedtime

Half of daily requirements (0.25 U/kg) used to construct PRE-MEAL sliding scales

Example: 60-kg patient requires 15 U/day of short-acting insulin
⇒ 5 U before each meal (when starting with a normal blood glucose)

Sample lispro (or regular insulin) sliding scale pre-meals:

Blood glucose	Insulin (U)
80–120	5
121–160	7
161–200	9
201–250	10
251–300	11
>300	Call house officer

FIGURE 5-2. Transitioning from intravenous insulin to subcutaneous insulin after closure of the anion gap: an example.

be $\sim$ 0.5 U/kg. Give half of this requirement as long-acting insulin (for example, 0.25 U/kg glargine at bedtime or split the long-acting dose as ⅔ NPH in the mornings and ⅓ NPH at bedtime). One-third of the remaining 0.25 U/kg dose should be used as the starting point for each of the pre-meal insulin sliding scales.

COMPLICATIONS

The mortality rate from DKA has declined in recent years. DKA is rarely fatal in patients < 45 years old. We recommend prophylactic anticoagulation to reduce the risk of arterial and venous thromboembolism, which likely result from dehydration and increased blood viscosity. Other less likely complications include cerebral edema, the acute respiratory distress syndrome, disseminated intravascular coagulation, pancreatitis, aspiration of gastric contents, pulmonary edema, and rhabdomyolysis.

REFERENCES

Textbook Chapters

Ennis ED, Stahl EJvB, Kreisberg RA. Diabetic ketoacidosis. In: Porte D Jr, Sherwin RS, editors. *Ellenberg & Rifkin's Diabetes Mellitus*. 5th ed. Connecticut: Appleton & Lange; 1997. pp. 827–844.

Review Articles

1. Chiasson JL, Aris-Jilwan N, Belanger R, et al. Diagnosis and treatment of diabetic ketoacidosis and the hyperglycemic hyperosmolar state. *CMAJ Canad Med Assoc J.* 2003;168:859–866.
2. Siperstein MD. Diabetic ketoacidosis and hyperosmolar coma. *Endoc & Metab Clin North Am.* 1992;21:415–432.

Epidemiology

Wetterhall SF, Olson DR, DeStefano F, et al. Trends in diabetes and diabetic complications, 1980–1987. *Diabetes Care*. 1992;15:960–967.

Diagnosis

Ennis ED, Stahl EjvB, Kreisberg RA. The hyperosmolar hyperglycemic syndrome. *Diabetes Rev*. 1994;1:115–126.

Pathogenesis and Treatment

Foster DW, McGarry JD. The metabolic derangements and treatment of diabetic ketoacidosis. *N Engl J Med*. 1991;6:495–502.

Gastroenterology

Acute Lower Gastrointestinal Bleed

KEY POINTS

General

1. Lower gastrointestinal (GI) bleed has a mortality rate of approximately 5%.
2. Diverticulosis is the most common cause of hematochezia.
3. Painless hematochezia suggests bleeding from diverticula or arteriovenous malformations (AVMs).
4. Bleeding with abdominal pain suggests ischemia, infection, or inflammation.
5. Fifteen percent of cases of hematochezia are due to an upper GI source.

Management

6. History and physical examination should focus on hemodynamic parameters and risk factors for upper or lower GI bleeding.
7. Laboratory testing should include a complete blood count, electrolytes, blood urea nitrogen, creatinine, type and cross, prothrombin time (PT), and activated partial thromboplastin time (PTT).
8. Barium studies of the upper and lower GI tract should be avoided.
9. A nasogastric lavage should be performed to rule out an upper GI source.

EGD

10. EGD should be performed if the NGL aspirate demonstrates gross blood, coffee grounds, or no blood and no bile.

11. EGD should also be considered in patients with massive hematochezia.
12. EGD should be performed if colonoscopy does not reveal a bleeding source.

Colonoscopy

13. Colonoscopy is the initial test of choice in patients with bilious, non-bloody nasogastric lavage aspirate who are hemodynamically stable.
14. Colonoscopy should be performed in patients with other nasogastric lavage results after EGD.

Angiography

15. Angiography is the initial test of choice if the rate of bleeding precludes pre-paration for colonoscopy due to hemo-dynamic instability.
16. Angiography should be performed if endoscopic evaluation cannot localize the site of bleeding, or if endoscopic therapy is unable to achieve hemostasis.
17. If the bleeding rate is low, and if the patient is hemodynamically stable, a tagged red blood cell scan should be performed before angiography.

DEFINITION

Lower gastrointestinal (GI) bleeding is defined as bleeding from a source distal to the Ligament of Treitz, most commonly, the colon.

Melena (the passage of black, tarry stools per rectum) is often associated with an upper GI but can occur in patients bleeding from a small bowel or proximal right colon source.

The passage of maroon stools is typical of a right colonic bleed, while the passage of bright red blood tends to occur with a left colon source. However, a patient may also pass bright red blood per rectum with a brisk upper GI bleed.

Hematochezia is responsible for roughly 20 hospitalizations per 100,000 adults, with a mortality rate of 3% to 5%, largely due to the higher incidence of lower GI bleeding in older patients with comorbidities.

In this chapter, we describe the approach for the patient presenting with moderate or severe hematochezia.

ETIOLOGY

A prospective study from 2001 assessed the relative frequencies of the various causes of severe hematochezia (Table 6-1). A colonic source was found in 81% of cases, an upper GI source in 15%, and a small bowel source in 1%. The remainder of cases did not have a source found on investigation. Other studies show slightly different ranges for patients with hematochezia (Table 6-2).

Diverticulosis is the most common cause of moderate to severe hematochezia, accounting for roughly one third of cases of brisk lower GI bleeds. The prevalence increases with age, from 30% at age 60 to 65% at age 85. Risk factors for diverticular bleeding include use of nonsteroidal anti-inflammatory drugs, constipation, and older age. Although diverticulosis usually occurs in the left colon, diverticula in the right colon account for the majority of cases of diverticular bleeding. The source of bleeding is arterial, and usually painless; some patients may experience mild abdominal cramping due to colonic spasm.

Colorectal Polyps and Cancer

Studies estimate that colorectal polyps and cancer account for roughly 20% of lower GI bleeds,

Table 6-1. Causes of Severe Hematochezia

Cause	Percent
Colon	
Diverticulosis	24.0
Internal hemorrhoids	11.3
Ischemic colitis	10.0
Rectal ulcers	7.4
Inflammatory bowel disease or other colitis	6.6
Post-polypectomy bleed	6.0
Colonic neoplasm	5.0
Colonic angiomas or radiation telangiectasias	4.6
Other	6.1
Total colon	**81.0**
Upper GI source (esophagus, stomach, duodenum)	15.3
Small bowel source	1.3
No source identified	2.4
Total non-colon	**19.0**
Total	**100.0**

Table 6-2. Causes of Hematochezia

Cause	Percent
Diverticulosis	17–40
Arteriovenous malformations	2–30
Colitis	9–21
Ischemic, infectious, radiation or inflammatory	10
Neoplasia, polyps, or post-polypectomy bleeding	11–14
Hemorrhoids, rectal varices	4–10
Upper GI source (proximal to Ligament of Treitz)	0–11
Small bowel source	2–9

slightly more if post-polypectomy bleeds are included as well. Colorectal polyps or cancer usually do not cause severe hematochezia, but rather, occult GI bleeding or intermittent mild hematochezia. Patients with colorectal cancer may have other associated signs and symptoms, including weight loss, constipation, or change in bowel habits. Bleeding results from erosions and ulcerations that develop from the friable mucosa. Although polyps may be removed endoscopically, treatment of colorectal cancer usually requires surgery.

Post-polypectomy bleeding may occur up to one week after the procedure, and is treated endoscopically.

Colitis

Inflammatory bowel disease and, in particular, ulcerative colitis, may present with hematochezia. Most patients will have other associated signs and symptoms, including abdominal pain, cramping and tenderness, fevers or chills, and increased white blood cell count.

Ischemic colitis typically presents with subjective pain out of proportion to physical findings. Moderate hematochezia usually occurs within 24 hours of pain onset.

The most common bacterial causes of hematochezia are Shigella, Campylobacter, Salmonella, and Enterohemorrhagic *E. coli*. *Clostridium difficile* infection may also cause hematochezia. In immunocompromised patients, cytomegalovirus infection should also be considered. Infectious colitis is unlikely to cause severe or massive bleeding.

Angiodysplasias

Angiodysplasias (also known as arteriovenous malformations, or AVMs) account for less than 10% of all cases of hematochezia, but may be the most common cause of lower GI bleeding in patients older than 65. Colonic AVMs are found in less than 1% of the population and are usually asymptomatic.

There is no need to treat AVMs found incidentally during a routine endoscopy or colonoscopy.

If found during an acute bleed, AVMs can be treated using cautery methods or argon plasma coagulation. Patients who experience recurrent bleeding from AVMs should be evaluated for angiodysplasia of the upper GI tract.

Miscellaneous Causes

Other causes of lower GI bleeding include radiation proctitis, hemorrhoids, solitary rectal ulcers, and colonic Dieulafoy's lesions.

Evaluation

History

The history should focus on determining risk factors for gastrointestinal hemorrhage, and assessing the severity and location of the bleed.

- Risk factors for upper GI bleeding:
  - History of *H. pylori* infection, or history of gastric or duodenal ulcers—may indicate peptic ulcer disease
  - Liver disease—may result in esophageal and gastric variceal bleeding
  - Use of nonsteroidal anti-inflammatory agents—may cause ulcerations anywhere throughout the gastrointestinal tract
- Risk factors for lower GI bleeding:
  - History of diverticulosis
  - Abdominal or pelvic radiation therapy, such as for prostate cancer—may indicate radiation colitis
  - Heart failure, atherosclerosis, recent low-flow states due to cardiovascular surgeries, etc.—may result in ischemic colitis
  - Family history of gastrointestinal cancers or disorders—may identify patients at higher risk of colorectal carcinoma or inflammatory bowel disease
- Location of bleeding:
  - Epigastric pain, hematemesis, melena, or hematochezia with hemodynamic

instability suggest the possibility of an upper GI source of bleeding.

- Maroon-colored stools suggest a small bowel or right-sided colon source, whereas bright red blood suggests a left-sided colon source.

- Other associated symptoms:
  - Fever, chills, and diarrhea suggest an infectious or inflammatory etiology.
  - Weight loss and change in bowel habits, with mild to moderate hematochezia in an older patient, may suggest a neoplasm.
  - Painless bleeding is associated with diverticulosis and angiodysplasia, whereas bleeding with abdominal pain or cramps may indicate an infectious, inflammatory, or ischemic cause.

- Severity of bleeding:
  - Orthostatic symptoms, chest pain, shortness of breath, palpitations, or lightheadedness should prompt urgent hemodynamic resuscitation and possibly cardiac evaluation in patients at higher risk for angina or myocardial infarction.

Physical Examination

- Orthostatic vital signs should be taken. A drop in blood pressure greater than 10 mm Hg or an increase in pulse greater than 10 bpm indicates blood loss of greater than 800 mL. Resting tachycardia or hypotension suggests blood loss greater than 1500 mL.

- Cardiovascular evaluation, including electrocardiogram (EKG), should be performed, as necessary.

- Abdominal examination should focus on identifying stigmata of chronic liver disease and any focal tenderness. If the history is unclear, a digital rectal examination should be performed to determine if the patient is passing maroon stools, bright red blood, or blood clots.

Initial Management

Please see Fig. 6-1 and Fig. 6-2 for an algorithmic approach to hematochezia.

Placement of two large-bore IV catheters, determination of hemodynamic status, and volume resuscitation (if necessary) should be

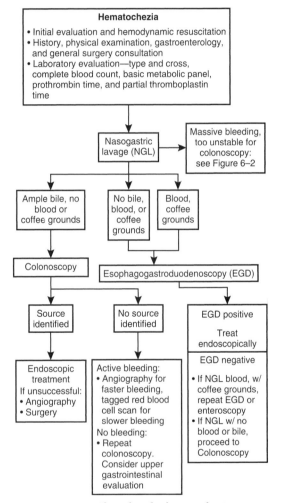

FIGURE 6–1. Algorithm for hematochezia.

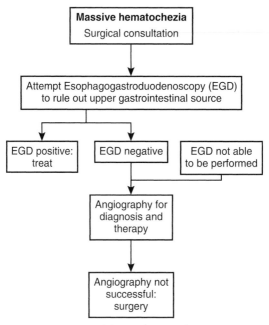

FIGURE 6–2. Massive hematochezia.

performed, and patients should be kept NPO. Gastroenterology and general surgery consultations should be requested. Laboratory testing should include:

- Type and cross for packed red blood cells, and, if necessary, platelets and fresh frozen plasma.
- Complete blood count: To determine hematocrit and rule out thrombocytopenia. The hematocrit may initially be normal, and may take 12–24 hr to reflect blood loss.
  - Hematocrit should be maintained around 30%.
  - Platelet count should be kept above 50,000/μL.
- Basic metabolic panel should be obtained. A BUN:Creatinine ratio greater than 20 should suggest the possibility of an upper GI source (although this may also be seen

in a patient with a "pre-renal" cause of acute renal failure).

- Prothrombin time (PT) and activated partial thromboplastin time (PTT): Presence of any coagulopathy should be corrected.
  - International Normalized Ratio (INR) > 1.5 should be corrected with fresh frozen plasma initially, and, if necessary(i.e., patients on Coumadin with supratherapeutic INR levels) Vitamin K_1, 10 mg given intravenously over 20–60 min.
- EKG and cardiac enzymes should be obtained in patients with risk factors for coronary artery disease.
- Nasogastric lavage should be performed in patients with hematochezia because up to 15% of patients have an upper gastrointestinal source of bleeding.
- Aspiration of blood or coffee-grounds confirms an upper GI source.
- Aspiration of clear fluid only, without bile, does not rule out an upper GI bleed because a duodenal bleeding source is not excluded.
- Aspiration of bilious fluid makes an upper GI source very unlikely. A false negative may occur if an intermittent bleed has stopped.

Radiologic Imaging

Plain films of the abdomen may be obtained to rule out complications, such as perforation, but have little role in the diagnosis and management of lower gastrointestinal bleeding.

In addition, use of barium studies may obscure visualization of a bleeding source during upper endoscopy or colonoscopy, and should not be performed.

DEFINITIVE MANAGEMENT

Nasogastric Lavage

If the nasogastric lavage is grossly bloody or contains coffee-grounds, an esophagogastroduodenoscopy (EGD) should be the initial procedure.

EGD should also be performed in patients with clear, nonbilious nasogastric aspirate, particularly in patients with risk factors for an upper GI bleed, because an upper GI source has not been ruled out.

If the nasogastric lavage demonstrates ample bile, without blood or coffee grounds, then a hemodynamically stable patient should be prepared for colonoscopy. Patients may be given 4 L of Golytely over 2 hours, either orally or through a nasogastric tube. Some physicians may also give metoclopramide, 10 mg IV single dose, to minimize nausea and vomiting and to expedite intestinal transit.

When to Perform EGD

EGD should be the initial test of choice:

- If the nasogastric lavage is grossly bloody or shows coffee grounds
- If the nasogastric lavage has no blood and no bile
- In a patient with massive lower GI bleeding, because a brisk upper GI bleed may present with profuse hematochezia

EGD should also be performed following a colonoscopy that does not demonstrate a potential or active bleeding source.

When to Perform Colonoscopy

Colonoscopy should be the initial test of choice in patients with a nasogastric lavage that shows bilious return without blood or coffee grounds.

- If the colonoscopy demonstrates a potentially treatable lesion, endoscopic therapy should be attempted. If treatment is unsuccessful and the bleeding continues, angiography (with or without preceding tagged red blood cell scan) should be performed (see following text).
- If the colonoscopy does not reveal a lesion and there is ongoing bleeding, angiography (with or without preceding tagged red blood cell scan) should be performed. If the bleeding has

ceased, a repeat colonoscopy may be attempted, followed by an upper GI evaluation if negative (see following text).

The diagnostic yield of colonoscopy for the diagnosis of lower GI bleeding is 69% to 80%. Prepped colonoscopy is preferred over unprepped colonoscopy, because the yield is higher, and the complication rate (such as perforations) is lower.

Colonoscopy is favored over angiography as the initial test of choice because colonoscopy has both a higher diagnostic yield and a lower rate of complications.

When to Perform Angiography

Angiography should be performed if:

- Massive hematochezia and the resulting hemodynamic instability warrant emergent intervention. In such cases, the two hours required for a colonoscopy prep may be unfeasible.
- Colonoscopy does not reveal a bleeding source because the rate of bleeding precludes adequate visualization.
- Attempted endoscopic therapy during colonoscopy is unsuccessful.

Angiography is able to visualize bleeding rates greater than 1 mL/min, although there have been reports of a positive angiography with bleeding rates as low as 0.4 mL/min.

In a stable patient, a bleeding scan (with 99m Tc-pertechnetate labeled red blood cells) is often performed before the angiography. Because the tagged red blood cell scan can detect bleeding rates of greater than 0.1 mL/min, angiography is unlikely to be positive if the tagged red blood cell scan is negative.

Surgery

If both endoscopic and angiographic therapies fail, surgery is the next option. An attempt to localize the site of bleeding is essential.

The morbidity and mortality rates, as well as the rebleeding rates for "blind" surgeries performed without adequate localization, is quite high.

Further Investigation

If colonoscopy, EGD, and angiography are unrevealing, a small bowel bleeding source should be suspected. Initial workup should include enteroscopy, followed by barium studies of the small bowel (such as a small bowel follow-through or enteroclysis). Capsule endoscopy may be considered in patients with negative barium studies.

REFERENCES

Textbook Chapters

Rockey DC. Gastrointestinal Bleeding. In: Feldman M, Friedman LS, and Sleisenger MH, editors, *Sleisenger and Fordtran's Gastrointestinal and Liver Disease*, 7th ed. Philadelphia. WB Saunders; 2002. pp. 226–232.

Practice Guidelines

1. Zuccaro Jr G. Management of the adult patient with acute lower gastrointestinal bleeding. *Am J Gastroent*. 1998;93:1202–1208.
2. Eisen GM, Dominitz JA, Faigel DO, et al. American Society for Gastrointestinal Endoscopy. Standards of Practice Committee. An annotated algorithmic approach to acute lower gastrointestinal bleeding. *Gastro Endosc*. 2001;53:859–863.
3. American Society for Gastrointestinal Endoscopy. The role of endoscopy in the patient with lower gastrointestinal bleeding. *Gastro Endosc*. 1998;48:685–688.

Epidemiology

Kovacs TOG, Jensen DM. Upper or small bowel hemorrhage that presents as hematochezia. *Tech Gastro Endosc*. 2001;3:206–215.

Diagnosis and Therapy

1. Jensen DM, Machicado GA. Colonoscopy for diagnosis and treatment of severe lower gastrointestinal bleeding. *Gastro Endosc Clin North Am.* 1997;7:477–498.
2. Cuellar RE, Gavaler JS, Alexander JA, et al. Gastrointestinal tract hemorrhage. The value of a nasogastric aspirate. *Arch Int Med.* 1990;150:1381–1384.
3. Gianfrancisco JA, Abcarian H. Pitfalls in the treatment of massive lower gastrointestinal bleeding with "blind" subtotal colectomy. *Dis Colon Rectum.* 1982;25:441–445.
4. Jensen DM. Diverticular bleeding: An appraisal based on stigmata of recent hemorrhage. *Tech Gastro Endosc.* 2001;192–198.

Figures 6-1 and 6-2

1. Rockey DC Gastrointestinal Bleeding. In: Feldman M, Friedman LS, and Sleisenger MH, editors, *Sleisenger and Fordtran's Gastrointestinal and Liver Disease,* 7th ed. Philadelphia. WB Saunders; 2002.
2. Zuccaro Jr G. Management of the adult patient with acute lower gastrointestinal bleeding. *Am J Gastroent.* 1998;93:1202–1208.
3. Eisen GM, Dominitz JA, Faigel DO, et al. American Society for Gastrointestinal Endoscopy. Standards of Practice Committee. An annotated algorithmic approach to acute lower gastrointestinal bleeding. *Gastro Endosc.* 2001;53:859–863.
4. American Society for Gastrointestinal Endoscopy. The role of endoscopy in the patient with lower gastrointestinal bleeding. *Gastro Endosc.* 1998;48:685–688.

Acute Pancreatitis

KEY POINTS

General

1. On admission, obtain:
   - Serum amylase and lipase. Levels three times the upper limit of normal are diagnostic.
   - Serum calcium and triglyceride levels to assess for hypercalcemia and hypertriglyceridemia as potential etiologies.
   - Right upper quadrant ultrasound to assess the biliary system and look for biliary stone disease.
2. Abdominal CT scanning should be performed in patients with severe acute pancreatitis (particularly those who deteriorate clinically) to assess for pancreatic necrosis.
3. Patients with gallstone pancreatitis should have a cholecystectomy during the current hospitalization if they are operative candidates. Patients who are poor surgical candidates should be offered endoscopic sphincterotomy.
4. Extensive workup for "idiopathic" pancreatitis should be reserved for older patients, patients with a family history of pancreatitis, patients with recurrent attacks, and patients with warning signs and symptoms of a serious underlying etiology (e.g., pancreatic neoplasms).

Severe Pancreatitis

5. On admission, aggressive fluid resuscitation with intensive care unit (ICU) monitoring is crucial. Six liters or more per

day are often required, and intravenous hydration at rates of 250 mL/hr or more should be initiated (lower infusion rates should be used in patients with renal or cardiac failure).

6. Sterile pancreatic necrosis should be medically managed. Prophylactic antibiotics (e.g., imipenem 500 mg IV every 8 hr) should not be routinely initiated in all patients with necrosis, but reserved for those with documented infected necrosis, signs and symptoms of sepsis, or the systemic inflammatory response syndrome (SIRS).

7. Patients with pancreatic necrosis who deteriorate clinically need urgent CT-guided needle aspiration of necrotic regions to assess for the presence of infected necrosis.

8. Patients with infected necrosis should receive antibiotics (imipenem or other appropriate enteric and anaerobic coverage) and surgical necrosectomy. Patients who are not surgical candidates can undergo percutaneous drainage by interventional radiology.

9. Endoscopic retrograde cholangiopancreatography (ERCP) within the first 24 to 72 hours in patients with gallstone pancreatitis and continued evidence of biliary obstruction, cholangitis or sepsis improves outcome in severe acute pancreatitis, but not mild pancreatitis.

DEFINITION

Acute pancreatitis is defined as inflammation of the exocrine pancreas with possible involvement of peripancreatic tissues and development of systemic complications.

INCIDENCE

Acute pancreatitis is common, with an incidence of 10 to 50 cases per 100,000 person-years. Although reports suggest a three-fold increase in incidence since the 1970s, this may reflect an increase in diagnosis rather than a true increase in disease burden.

Patients with HIV have a higher incidence of acute pancreatitis. Acute pancreatitis is also more common in women, who usually develop gallstone pancreatitis. Men are more likely to have alcohol-induced pancreatitis. Gallstone disease and alcohol use account for approximately 70% to 80% of cases of pancreatitis. Ten percent of cases are due to other diagnosable factors, and the remaining 10% are "idiopathic." (See Table 7-1.)

MORBIDITY AND MORTALITY

Acute pancreatitis spontaneously resolves in 75% to 85% of cases. The remaining cases tend to follow a more severe course, with both local and systemic complications. Mortality within the first two weeks is due to the systemic inflammatory response syndrome and organ failure. Mortality after the first 2 weeks is usually due to infectious complications and sepsis.

The overall mortality for acute pancreatitis is approximately 10%, but this number represents a heterogeneous group of patients. Interstitial pancreatitis has a 1.5% mortality, pancreatitis complicated by sterile necrosis has a 12% to 14% mortality, and pancreatitis with infected necrosis has a mortality rate as high as 30%.

Patients with their first episode of acute pancreatitis have a higher likelihood of morbidity and mortality. Obesity is associated with a worse prognosis, as more peripancreatic fat leads to greater risk and degree of necrosis. In fact, 66% of obese patients have severe pancreatitis

Table 7-1. Causes of Acute Pancreatitis

Cause	Useful tests
Gallstones	RUQ ultrasound, ALT > 3 times normal
Alcohol use	Medical history, lipase: amylase ratio > 2
Hypertriglyceridemia	Lipid profile on admission
Hypercalcemia	Calcium level on admission
Biliary sludge, microlithiasis	EUS, biliary crystal analysis
Medications (see Box 7-1)	Medical history
Infections	Signs and symptoms consistent with infectious etiology
Post-ERCP	Medical history, amylase, and lipase > 5 times normal 4 hr after procedure

Trauma or postoperative	
Pancreas divisum	CT, MRCP, EUS, ERCP
Choledochal cyst	MRCP, ERCP
Duodenal disease: Crohn's disease, ulcers	EGD with possible biopsies
Ischemia: Vasculitis, shock	

Genetic diseases	
Hereditary pancreatitis	Genetic testing for cationic trypsinogen mutation
Cystic fibrosis	Genetic testing
Autoimmune pancreatitis	IgG4 level

RUQ = right upper quadrant, ALT = alanine aminotransferase, EUS = endoscopic ultrasound, MRCP = magnetic resonance cholangiopancreatography, ERCP = endoscopic retrograde cholangiopancreatography, EGD = esophagogastroduodenoscopy.

Box 7-1. Medications Causing Acute Pancreatitis

HIV therapy

- Didanosine
- Pentamidine

Immunosuppressive medications

- Azathioprine
- 6-mercaptopurine

Antimicrobials

- Sulfonamides
- Isoniazid
- Tetracycline
- Metronidazole
- Erythromycin
- Nitrofurantoin

Cardiac Medications

- Angiotensin-converting enzyme inhibitors
- Furosemide
- Methyldopa

Miscellaneous

- Salicylates
- Valproic acid
- Estrogens
- Cimetidine
- Ranitidine
- Sulindac
- Acetaminophen

(with 36% mortality) compared with 6% of non-obese patients.

Roughly, 80% of deaths from pancreatitis are due to complications, with 60% of deaths occurring in the first week, usually due to systemic complications (primarily pulmonary), and 40% of deaths occurring after the first week, primarily due to sepsis. Infected necrosis causes death later in the disease course.

ETIOLOGY

We will briefly discuss a few of the more common causes of acute pancreatitis. Please refer to Table 7-1 for a listing of etiologies of acute pancreatitis.

Gallstones

Gallstone pancreatitis accounts for 35% of acute pancreatitis. Only 3% to 7% of patients with gallstones develop acute pancreatitis. The risk of pancreatitis is inversely proportional to stone size, with stones smaller than 5 mm having the highest risk. Although the risk of developing gallstone pancreatitis is higher in men with cholelithiasis, gallstone pancreatitis is more common in women because more women have gallstones.

Patients often present with a history of biliary colic prior to the development of pancreatitis. Alanine aminotransferase (ALT) greater than three times the upper limit of normal in a patient with pancreatitis is highly suggestive of gallstone pancreatitis (ALT > 150 IU/L has a 95% positive predictive value for gallstone pancreatitis).

Treatment is cholecystectomy, preferably during the same hospitalization.

Alcohol

Alcohol-induced pancreatitis is more common in men and occurs in 10% of persons who are chronic alcoholics. Most cases of alcohol-induced pancreatitis occur in patients with chronic pancreatitis.

Patients with alcohol-induced pancreatitis should be advised to abstain from alcohol intake.

Hypertriglyceridemia

Hypertriglyceridemia causes less than 4% of cases of acute pancreatitis. Triglyceride levels greater than 1000 mg/dL are required to induce disease. The most common types of familial hyperlipidemia associated with acute pancreatitis are Type V (40%), Type I (35%), and Type II (15%). In adults, such high triglyceride levels are usually caused by a combination of an inherited familial hyperlipidemia syndrome and an acquired etiology of hypertriglyceridemia, such as obesity, diabetes mellitus, or use of medications.

The three common presentations of hypertriglyceridemia-induced pancreatitis are:

- Poorly controlled diabetes with hypertriglyceridemia
- Alcoholism with hypertriglyceridemia
- Drug or diet-induced hypertriglyceridemia in a nondiabetic, nonalcoholic and nonobese patient.

Trigylceride levels should be obtained on admission. If triglyceride levels are checked after the patient has been fasting for a period of time, the results may be falsely low. Amylase levels may be falsely normal in the presence of hypertriglyceridemia because the high triglyceride levels interfere with the amylase assay.

Hypercalcemia

Hypercalcemia is an uncommon cause of acute pancreatitis. The association of hyperparathyroidism with pancreatitis is debatable. Less than 0.5% of cases of acute pancreatitis are due to hyperparathyroidism, and fewer than 1.5% of patients with hyperparathyroidism develop acute pancreatitis.

Medications

Medication-induced pancreatitis (see Box 7-1) accounts for 1.4% of cases of pancreatitis, and may be due to either dose-dependent effects or idiosyncratic reactions.

Infections

Various infectious agents may cause pancreatitis (Box 7-2), and the key to diagnosis is to recognize the associated symptoms and signs.

Patients with HIV infection are at a higher risk for development of acute pancreatitis due to either medication side effects or infectious etiologies.

Box 7-2. Infectious Causes of Acute Pancreatitis

Parasites

- Ascaris
- Clonorchis
- Toxoplasma
- Cryptosporidium

Viruses

- Coxsackievirus
- Mumps
- Cytomegalovirus
- Hepatitis B virus
- Varicella zoster virus
- Herpes simplex virus

Bacteria

- Tuberculosis
- *Mycobacterium avium* complex
- Mycoplasma
- Legionella
- Leptospira
- Salmonella

Fungi

- Aspergillus

Post-ERCP

Acute pancreatitis is a potential complication of endoscopic retrograde cholangiopancreatography (ERCP), occurring in 3% of diagnostic and 5% of therapeutic ERCPs, and up to 25% of ERCPs performed for Sphincter of Oddi manometry. Risk factors for development of acute pancreatitis after ERCP are:

- Female sex
- Younger age
- Prior history of post-ERCP pancreatitis
- Sphincter of Oddi dysfunction
- Pancreas divisum
- Common bile duct smaller than 5 mm
- Difficult cannulation
- Pancreatic duct injection
- Precut sphincterotomy

A high index of suspicion for post-ERCP pancreatitis should be maintained for patients with one or more risk factors.

Up to 70% of patients will have asymptomatic amylase elevations after ERCP. Amylase level less than 276 U/L and lipase level less than 1000 U/L have a negative predictive value for post-ERCP pancreatitis of 97%. An amylase level of greater than five times the upper limit of normal 4 hours after ERCP in an appropriate clinical setting is highly suggestive of pancreatitis. Serum trypsinogen 2 levels greater than three times the upper limit of normal 6 hours after ERCP may accurately indicate pancreatitis, but availability limits its use.

Miscellaneous Causes

Other uncommon causes of acute pancreatitis include biliary sludge or microlithiasis, hereditary pancreatitis, cystic fibrosis, and vasculitides.

In biliary sludge and microlithiasis, microscopic analysis of biliary secretions reveals the presence of cholesterol or bilirubinate crystals.

Subsequent cholecystectomy, endoscopic sphincterotomy, or ursodeoxycholic acid therapy may reduce recurrent episodes of acute pancreatitis in these patients.

DETERMINING THE ETIOLOGY OF ACUTE PANCREATITIS

The approach to determining the etiology of acute pancreatitis is outlined in Fig. 7-1. A thorough analysis is beyond the scope of this chapter, but a brief discussion is presented here.

On presentation, a thorough history and physical examination should be performed, any risk factors identified and pursued, and all medications reviewed. Initial workup should include a right upper quadrant ultrasound, admission triglyceride and calcium levels and other laboratory tests as suggested by the history and physical examination.

If no cause is identified and the patient is a young, otherwise healthy individual with no warning signs (weight loss, anemia, malaise) suggestive of a more serious disease, and no family history of acute pancreatitis, further workup may be deferred until the second attack. Many such patients have an isolated episode of pancreatitis without recurrence.

However, in older patients, patients with worrisome signs and symptoms, or patients with recurrent acute pancreatitis, further evaluation is warranted. Initial investigation should begin with an abdominal CT scan, looking for the presence of a cystic or solid pancreatic neoplasm, ampullary tumors, evidence of chronic pancreatitis, or anatomic variations. Following the CT scan, an endoscopic ultrasound (EUS) may be performed to assess for microlithiasis, abnormal biliary anatomy, intraductal papillary mucinous tumors, and chronic pancreatitis. EUS provides the opportunity for fine needle aspiration of any suspected neoplasms. EUS has been shown in one study to reveal the cause of pancreatitis in 68% of patients with "idiopathic" acute pancreatitis.

First episode of acute pancreatitis:

- Review medications for potential etiology
- Thorough history and physical examination
  for possible causes (see Table 7-1)
- Initial workup:
  - Gallstone disease—right upper quadrant ultrasound
  - Alcohol use—history, obtain blood alcohol level
  - Hypertriglyceridemia—admission serum lipid profile
  - Hypercalcemia—admission serum calcium

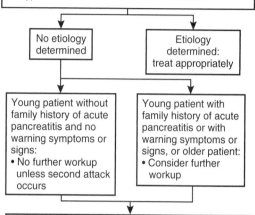

No etiology
determined

Etiology
determined:
treat appropriately

Young patient without
family history of acute
pancreatitis and no
warning symptoms or
signs:
- No further workup
  unless second attack
  occurs

Young patient with
family history of acute
pancreatitis or with
warning symptoms or
signs, or older patient:
- Consider further
  workup

Step 1:
Abdominal CT scan: Assess for chronic pancreatitis,
cystic or solid pancreatic neoplasms, ampullary
tumors.
Endoscopic ultrasound: Assess for biliary sludge,
cystic or solid pancreatic neoplasms, abnormal
biliary anatomy (choledochal cysts, pancreas
divisum, etc.), intraductal papillary mucinous tumor,
chronic pancreatitis.
Step 2:
If no etiology found, proceed with magnetic
resonance cholangiopancreatography or endoscopic
retrograde cholangiopancreatography to assess for
pancreatic duct strictures, ampullary stenoses,
possible Sphincter of Oddi dysfunction.
Step 3:
Consider empiric treatment for biliary sludge or
microlithiasis with cholecystectomy. If patient is a
poor operative candidate, consider endoscopic
sphincterotomy or ursodeoxycholic acid therapy.
Step 4:
Consider less likely etiologies, such as:
- Autoimmune pancreatitis—send total IgG and
  IgG4 levels
- Consider genetic testing for hereditary pancreatitis
  or cystic fibrosis.

FIGURE 7–1. Determining the etiology of acute pancreatitis.

If no cause is identified, many gastroenterologists proceed with biliary imaging, via either magnetic resonance cholangiopancreatography (MRCP) or ERCP. If no etiology is found, empiric cholecystectomy (or endoscopic sphincterotomy) for biliary sludge or microlithiasis is reasonable. If attacks recur, further evaluation for autoimmune pancreatitis, hereditary pancreatitis, or cystic fibrosis may be performed.

CLINICAL FEATURES

Patients usually relate a history of epigastric pain, sometimes with radiation to the back, or in association with left upper quadrant pain. The pain may follow a large meal in cases of gallstone pancreatitis, or may follow alcohol use by 1 to 3 days in alcohol-induced pancreatitis.

The pain usually has a violent onset that follows a crescendo pattern, with a time to maximal pain of 10 to 30 minutes, and is almost always associated with significant nausea and vomiting. Patients may note some relief of their pain with bending forward at the waist and may report anorexia.

Physical examination reveals tachycardia, tachypnea, and fever, and in cases of gallstone pancreatitis, icteric sclera may be noted. Respiratory distress may be present, due to pleural effusions or acute respiratory distress syndrome (ARDS). Although dramatic, Cullen's sign (ecchymoses of the peri-umbilical region) and Grey-Turner's signs (ecchymoses of the flank region) are uncommonly seen. Their presence indicates retroperitoneal bleeding due to hemorrhage complicating pancreatic necrosis. An ileus occurs in 25% of cases of interstitial pancreatitis but 95% of cases of necrotizing pancreatitis.

DIAGNOSIS

Laboratory Testing

Aside from the history and physical examination, diagnosis of acute pancreatitis relies on elevations in serum amylase and lipase.

Amylase has a half-life of approximately 10 hours, peaks within 12 hours, and may be normal in 24 hours if no additional amylase spillage occurs. Amylase levels greater than threefold normal are usually diagnostic of acute pancreatitis. Elevated amylase levels are sensitive but not specific for the diagnosis of pancreatitis because many other conditions may cause high amylase levels (Box 7-3). Lower amylase levels are found in alcoholic pancreatitis, and levels may be normal in acute pancreatitis secondary to hyperlipidemia. Amylase levels correlate well with the clinical course.

Lipase remains elevated longer than amylase, and when levels greater than threefold normal are used for diagnosis of pancreatitis, lipase has a sensitivity and specificity of about 99%.

Box 7-3. Other Causes of Elevated Amylase Levels

- Macromylasemia—decreased renal clearance of protein-bound amylase leads to increased amylase levels without clinical pancreatitis
- Acute or chronic renal failure
- Salivary gland disease
- Gastrointestinal diseases
  - Cholecystitis
  - Intestinal obstruction
  - Intestinal perforation
  - Intestinal ischemia or infarction
- Gynecological diseases
  - Ruptured ectopic pregnancy
  - Salpingitis

The lipase-to-amylase ratio may help to distinguish gallstone-induced pancreatitis from alcoholic pancreatitis. Gallstones cause higher increases in amylase, and alcohol causes higher increases in lipase. A lipase-to-amylase ratio > 2 has 91% sensitivity and 76% specificity for alcoholic pancreatitis, and a ratio > 5 has 31% sensitivity and close to 100% specificity for alcoholic pancreatitis. Increased ALT to 3 times normal is highly specific to gallstone pancreatitis.

Measurement of both serum amylase and lipase increases specificity as compared to either test alone but does not significantly improve sensitivity.

Imaging

A right upper quadrant ultrasound should be performed in all patients admitted for acute pancreatitis. Ultrasound imaging is a poor modality for diagnosing acute pancreatitis but is very useful for assessing the presence of biliary stone disease as the etiological factor for pancreatitis.

Plain films of the abdomen are useful to rule out other potential diagnoses, such as intestinal perforation or obstruction. The plain film may also show a "sentinel loop" or "colon cutoff sign" suggesting acute pancreatitis. A sentinel loop is an ileus in a segment of small bowel, and the colon cutoff sign is caused by lack of air distal to the splenic flexure due to colonic spasm from pancreatic inflammation. Severe acute pancreatitis may cause a generalized ileus visible on plain abdominal films.

Chest x-ray may reveal potential causes of respiratory compromise, such as pleural effusions, atelectasis, or, in severe cases, acute respiratory distress syndrome.

Abdominal CT scan should be used to determine the severity and presence of complications of acute pancreatitis, particularly pancreatic necrosis or fluid collections.

Assessment of Severity

Two scoring systems are commonly used to identify patients with severe pancreatitis who have an increased risk of complications: Ranson's criteria (Table 7-2) and APACHE II. A Ranson score > 3 or an APACHE II score > 8 indicates severe pancreatitis. Limitations of Ranson's criteria include a 48-hour time requirement for score determination, and a lack of ability to reassess severity at later points during the hospitalization. The APACHE II scoring system

Table 7-2. Ranson's Criteria

Gallstone Pancreatitis

On admission	After 48 hours
Age > 70 years	Decrease in hematocrit > 10%
WBC > 18,000/µL	Increase in BUN > 2 mg/dL
Glucose > 220 mg/dL	Serum calcium < 8 mg/dL
LDH > 400 U/L	Base deficit > 5 mmol/L
AST > 250 U/L	Fluid deficit > 4 L

Nongallstone Pancreatitis

On admission	After 48 hours
Age > 55 years	Decrease in hematocrit > 10%
WBC > 16,000/µL	Increase in BUN > 5 mg/dL
Glucose > 200 mg/dL	Serum calcium < 8 mg/dL
LDH > 350 U/L	PaO_2 < 60 mmHg
AST > 250 U/L	Base deficit > 4 mmol/L
	Fluid deficit > 6 L

Base deficit = (actual pH − predicted pH) × 67

allows determination of severity on admission
and at any point during the hospital course;
however, complexity of scoring may limit
its use.

Hemoconcentration (hematocrit greater than
44%) on admission and lack of normalization at
24 hours after admission appear to be good
predictors of severe pancreatitis. This scoring
system offers a quick and simple method for
assessment of severity.

Contrast-enhanced abdominal CT scan
results may also correlate with severity. Lack of
enhancement of greater than one third of the
pancreas is associated with severe pancreatitis
and increased risk for infected necrosis. One
caveat is that a CT scan performed too early may
underestimate the disease course.

TREATMENT

Mild Acute Pancreatitis

Patients with mild, or interstitial, pancreatitis
(without necrosis) may be treated conservatively
with intravenous hydration, analgesia, and
NPO status. Although morphine has been mal-
igned due to its effect in Sphincter of Oddi
pressure, no clinical evidence suggests that
morphine worsens the course of acute pancreatitis. Fentanyl or other opiate analgesics may
be safely used in patients with acute pancreatitis. We discourage meperidine because the
risk of adverse events outweigh the theoretical
benefits.

Most patients will improve within one week.
Further therapy should target the precipitating
factors. Patients with pancreatitis due to gallstone disease should be offered a cholecystectomy during the hospitalization. Patients suffering
from chronic excessive alcohol use should be
offered information on substance abuse cessation
programs.

Severe Acute Pancreatitis—General Principles

Supportive Care

Hemodynamic monitoring and fluid resuscitation are critical in the therapy of severe pancreatitis. At least 4 to 6 L (and often more) of fluid per day are required initially, given at rates of 250 mL/hr or greater. Insufficient repletion may increase the risk of developing pancreatic necrosis. Monitoring of urine output, oxygen saturation, and hemodynamic variables, preferably in an intensive care unit (ICU) setting, will help to guide resuscitation.

Nutrition

Supplemental nutrition should be initiated in patients who are expected to maintain NPO status for greater than one week. Studies comparing jejunal feeding of an elemental diet versus total parenteral nutrition (TPN) demonstrated that patients given jejunal feeding:

- Developed fewer total and septic complications
- Had an insignificant decrease in disease severity (this study may have been underpowered to show a significant difference)
- Showed statistically significant improvement in levels of acute phase reactants and disease severity scores

In addition, jejunal feeding was less expensive than TPN, and associated with a lower incidence of infection, shorter duration of hospitalization, and reduced need for surgical intervention.

Thus, patients with severe acute pancreatitis who will not resume oral intake within 7 days should be started on elemental jejunal feedings, preferably within 48 hours of admission.

Refeeding

Patients with acute pancreatitis should not be offered oral feeling unless:

- All major complications have been successfully treated
- Patient is pain free without the use of analgesic medications
- Serum amylase or lipase levels are within normal limits

The risk of recurrent pain in patients beginning oral feeding is greatest in the first 48 hours, and is associated with:

- Necrotizing pancreatitis
- Serum lipase levels more than three times the upper limit of normal one day prior to refeeding
- Having pain for a longer period of time prior to refeeding

Refeeding should begin with clear liquids and advanced to a regular diet within 4 to 5 days.

Severe Acute Pancreatitis—Complications

Systemic Complications

Death within the first 2 weeks is usually due to systemic complications and organ failure. Shock is the most important and deadly complication within the first 48 hours, and results from intravascular fluid shifts into the gastrointestinal tract, retroperitoneum, and peritoneum. In addition, cytokine-induced myocardial depression contributes to cardiovascular compromise. As previously discussed, aggressive volume resuscitation, and perhaps use of pressor agents, should be pursued in an ICU setting with hemodynamic monitoring.

Hypomagnesemia and hypocalcemia may also occur. For those patients with hypomagnesemia, magnesium repletion should be instituted.

Calcium should only be repleted if the patient shows signs and symptoms of hypocalcemia.

Pulmonary Complications

Respiratory compromise may be due to pleural effusions, atelectasis, or acute respiratory distress syndrome (ARDS). Pulmonary complications tend to occur between days 3 to 7 in the disease course, with up to 10% of patients requiring mechanical ventilation. The development of respiratory failure is associated with up to 50% mortality. A discussion of the management of pleural effusions and ARDS is beyond the scope of this chapter.

Renal Complications

Hypovolemia and hypotension may result in acute renal failure, either due to "pre-renal" causes or acute tubular necrosis. Renal failure occurs within the first week, usually in conjunction with other systemic complications. The presence of renal failure increases mortality by up to 50%, an indication of the severity of the underlying illness. With supportive care, renal failure is potentially reversible as the pancreatitis and accompanying systemic inflammatory response syndrome resolve. Close hemodynamic monitoring is indicated during fluid resuscitation to avoid volume overload and pulmonary edema.

Pancreas

Pancreatic necrosis is a potentially fatal complication of acute pancreatitis. Patients with infected necrosis have a mortality rate as high as 30%. Although infection may occur early during the course of the disease, most cases occur after the first week. One series showed a 24% infection rate of pancreatic necrosis in week one and a 71% infection rate in week three. The major organisms are enteric gram-negative bacteria, including *Escherichia coli, Pseudomonas,* and *Klebsiella.* Infection with fungi or gram-positive bacteria usually occurs in patients receiving prophylactic antibiotics. Seventy-five percent of infections are monomicrobial.

Patients with sterile necrosis should be medically managed with nutritional and other supportive care as needed, and surgical intervention should be avoided. The use of prophylactic antibiotics in patients with sterile necrosis is controversial:

- Earlier studies and two meta-analyses (one with eight trials, the other with four trials), demonstrated reduction in morbidity and mortality.
- A recent prospective randomized controlled trial using placebo or ciprofloxacin and metronidazole did not show any mortality benefit or reduction in the development of infected necrosis. However, this study was powered to show a 20% absolute difference. Therefore, smaller degrees of benefit may have been missed. Also, patients who developed signs of sepsis or SIRS were switched to open-label antibiotics; thus, the study results may not apply to this population.

It is reasonable to reserve use of prophylactic antibiotics for patients who show signs of clinical deterioration, or those who develop sepsis or SIRS. Imipenem or other enteric and anaerobic coverage (such as ciprofloxacin with metronidazole) may be used. Patients receiving prophylactic antibiotics who show evidence of deterioration should be assessed for fungal or gram-positive bacterial infection. If the patient does not begin to improve within one week, or worsens clinically, a CT-guided needle aspiration of necrotic areas should be performed to rule out infected necrosis.

Once infected necrosis develops, surgical debridement is the treatment of choice, and antibiotics should be initiated. Although some studies have shown successful treatment of patients with percutaneous drainage, these methods are best reserved for patients who are too ill to tolerate surgery, or, because of comorbid conditions, are poor operative candidates.

A summary of the therapeutic approach to acute pancreatitis is presented in Fig. 7-2.

Gallstone Pancreatitis

Evidence shows that early ERCP (within 24–72 hr) for patients with biliary obstruction and severe acute pancreatitis decreases the complication rate and incidence of biliary sepsis from 12% in untreated patients to 0% in treated

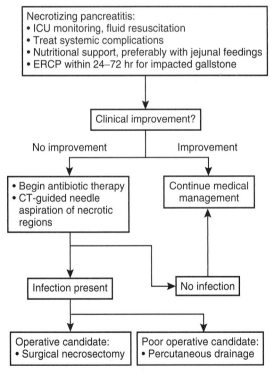

FIGURE 7–2. Therapeutic approach to acute pancreatitis. ICU = intensive care unit, ERCP = endoscopic retrograde cholangiopancreatography.

patients. However, ERCP is no better than medical management in patients without biliary obstruction. Similarly, no benefit was noted with early ERCP in patients with mild acute pancreatitis. With this in mind, the approach to patients with severe gallstone-induced acute pancreatitis follows:

- Patients with elevated liver function tests (LFTs) or radiographic findings suggestive of gallstone-induced pancreatitis should be assessed for the presence of cholangitis.
- If cholangitis is present (fevers, right upper quadrant pain, and jaundice, with increased white blood cell count), ERCP should be performed urgently.
- If cholangitis is absent, LFTs should be rechecked within 12 hr:
  □ If LFTs are increasing → proceed to ERCP.
  □ If LFTs are decreasing slowly → consider MRCP to rule out common duct stones, reserving ERCP for patients with documented common duct stones.
  □ If LFTs are decreasing rapidly → consider intraoperative cholangiogram or preoperative MRCP to assess for retained common duct stones.

REFERENCES

Textbook Chapter

DiMagno EP, Chari S. Acute Pancreatitis. In: Feldman M, Friedman LS, and Sleisenger MH, editors. *Sleisenger and Fordtran's Gastrointestinal and Liver Disease,* 7th ed. Philadelphia. WB Saunders; 2002, pp. 913–942.

Review Article

Swaroop VS, Chari ST, Clain JE. Severe acute pancreatitis. *JAMA* 2004;291:2865–2868.

Diagnosis

1. Papachristou GI, Whitcomb DC. Predictors of severity and necrosis in acute pancreatitis. *Gastro Clin North Am*. 2004;33:871–890.
2. Yadav D, Agarwal N, Pitchumoni CS. A critical evaluation of laboratory tests in acute pancreatitis. *Am J Gastro*. 2002;97:1309–1318.
3. Draganov P, Forsmark CE. "Idiopathic" pancreatitis. *Gastroenterology* 2005;128: 756–763.

Treatment

1. Werner J, Feuerbach S, Uhl W, et al. Management of acute pancreatitis: From surgery to interventional intensive care. *Gut* 2005;54:426–436.
2. Mayerle J, Simon P, Merch MM. Medical treatment of acute pancreatitis. *Gastroenterol Clin North Am*. 2004;33:855–869.
3. Tenner S. Initial management of acute pancreatitis: Critical issues during the first 72 hours. *Am J Gastro*. 2004;99:2489–2494.
4. Isenmann R, Runzi M, Kron M, et al. Prophylactic antibiotic treatment in patients with predicted severe acute pancreatitis: A placebo-controlled, double-blind trial. *Gastroenterology* 2004;126:997–1004.
5. Ayub K, Imada R, Slavin J. Endoscopic retrograde cholangiopancreatography in gallstone-associated acute pancreatitis. *Coch Data System Rev*. 2005; 2.

Acute Upper Gastrointestinal Bleed

KEY POINTS

General

1. Acute upper gastrointestinal (GI) bleed has a mortality rate of approximately 10%.
2. Gastroduodenal ulcers are the most common cause of acute upper GI bleeding.
3. Gastroesophageal variceal hemorrhage is common in patients with cirrhosis and has a high mortality rate.

Management

4. History and physical examination should focus on hemodynamic parameters and risk factors for upper GI bleeding.
5. Laboratory testing should include a complete blood count, electrolytes, blood urea nitrogen, creatinine, type and cross, prothrombin time (PT), and activated partial thromboplastin time (PTT).
6. Barium studies of the upper and lower GI tract should be avoided.
7. Use of nasogastric lavage erythromycin (1–3 mg/kg IV) or metoclopramide (10 mg IV) may improve endoscopic visualization.
8. High-dose proton pump inhibitors should be started. Octreotide should be administered if the patient has findings suggestive of cirrhosis.
9. Angiography or surgery should be considered for ulcer hemorrhage refractory to maximal medical and endoscopic therapy.

10. Transjugular intrahepatic portosystemic shunt (TIPS) placement should be considered for esophageal variceal bleeding, refractory to maximal medical and endoscopic therapy, or for isolated gastric variceal bleeding.

DEFINITION

Upper gastrointestinal (GI) bleeding is defined as bleeding from a source proximal to the Ligament of Treitz. Melena, the passage of black, tarry stools per rectum, is often associated with an upper GI bleed. However, melena may occur in patients with a small bowel or proximal right-sided colon bleeding source. Patients can pass bright red blood per rectum with a brisk upper GI bleed.

Upper GI bleeding occurs five times more often than lower GI bleeding, and is more common in male and elderly patients.

There are 400,000 hospitalizations annually in the United States for upper GI bleeding Despite advances in therapy, the mortality rate for upper GI bleeding ranges from 4% to 14%, largely due to the higher mortality rate in elderly patients with numerous serious comorbidities (30%–44% of upper GI bleeding occurs in patients over the age of 65). Mortality from upper GI bleeding is 0.4% in patients under the age of 60 and rises to 11% in patients over the age of 80.

The major causes of upper GI bleeding are gastric and duodenal ulcers, esophageal varices, and Mallory-Weiss tears. Other less common causes are Dieulafoy's lesions (an arterial branch protruding through a mucosal defect, most commonly found in the gastric fundus), arteriovenous malformations, esophagitis, and neoplasms (Box 8-1).

Box 8-1. Causes of Acute Upper GI Bleeding

Common

Gastroduodenal ulcer
Esophageal varices
Mallory-Weiss tear

Less Common

Dieulafoy's lesions
Vascular ectasia
Portal hypertensive gastropathy
Gastric antral vascular ectasia
Neoplasia
Esophagitis
Gastric erosions

Infrequent

Esophageal ulcers
Erosive duodenitis
Aortoenteric fistula
Hemobilia
Pancreatic source
Crohn's disease

Rockey DC. Gastrointestinal Bleeding. In: Feldman M, Friedman LS, and Sleisenger MH, editors. *Sleisenger and Fordtran's Gastrointestinal and Liver Disease,* 7th ed. Philadelphia. WB Saunders; 2002. p. 215. Reproduced with permission, 2005.

INITIAL EVALUATION

History

The history should focus on determining risk factors and potential etiologies for gastrointestinal hemorrhage, and assessment of rebleeding risk. In addition, potential complications due to coexisting medical conditions (such as myocardial ischemia in patients with coronary artery disease) should also be evaluated.

- Potential etiologies:
  - *Helicobacter pylori* infection or history of gastric or duodenal ulcers

- ○ Nonsteroidal anti-inflammatory drug (NSAID) use
- ○ Liver disease: potential sources include esophageal or gastric varices. Portal hypertensive gastropathy and gastric antral vascular ectasia usually do not present with acute upper GI bleeding.
- ○ Nausea and vomiting prior to hematemesis suggest Mallory-Weiss tears as a potential etiology.
- ○ Weight loss or anorexia may suggest malignancy.

Rebleeding risk is highest in elderly patients with many comorbidities, and those with persistent hypotension, hematemesis, or hematochezia (Box 8-2). There are many prognostic scoring systems, but their overall reliability remains low.

Physical Examination

- Orthostatic vital signs should be taken. A drop in blood pressure greater than

Box 8-2. Risk Factors for Rebleeding and Prognostic Variables

- Age > 60
- Severe or numerous comorbidities, such as coronary artery disease, renal failure, congestive heart failure, or cirrhosis
- Hypotension or shock at presentation
- Requiring ≥ 6 units of packed red blood cells
- Coagulopathy
- Red blood on nasogastric lavage, hematemesis, or hematochezia
- Bleeding or rebleeding occurring during hospitalization
- Presence of a high-risk lesion on endoscopy, such as arterial bleeding, visible vessel, or clot

10 mmHg or an increase in pulse greater than 10 bpm indicates blood loss of greater than 800 mL. Resting tachycardia or hypotension suggests blood loss greater than 1500 mL.

- Cardiovascular evaluation, including electrocardiogram (EKG), should be performed, as necessary.
- Abdominal examination should focus on identifying stigmata of chronic liver disease and any focal tenderness. Digital rectal examination should be performed.

INITIAL MANAGEMENT

See Fig. 8-1 and Fig. 8-2 for an algorithmic approach to acute upper GI bleeding, with details for gastroduodenal ulcer and gastroesophageal variceal hemorrhage.

Hemodynamically stable patients with acute upper GI bleeding may be managed in a telemetry unit, whereas those with hemodynamic instability or persistent bleeding should be admitted to the intensive care unit.

Placement of two large-bore IV catheters, determination of hemodynamic status, and volume resuscitation (if necessary) should be performed, and patients should be kept NPO. Laboratory testing should include:

- Type and cross for packed red blood cells, and, if necessary, platelets and fresh frozen plasma.
- Complete blood count: To determine hematocrit and rule out thrombocytopenia. The hematocrit may initially be normal, and may take 12–24 hr to reflect blood loss.
  - Hematocrit should be maintained around 30%. In patients with esophageal variceal hemorrhage, the hematocrit should not exceed 30%. At higher hematocrit levels, portal pressure will rise and increase the risk of rebleeding.

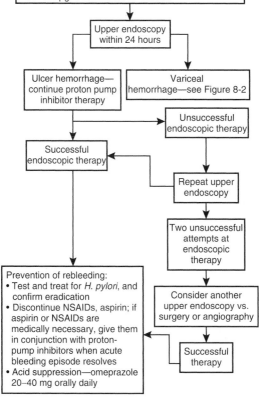

Upper GI bleeding
- Initial evaluation and hemodynamic resuscitation
- History, physical examination, gastroenterology consultation
- Laboratory evaluation—type and cross, CBC, basic metabolic panel (sodium, potassium, chloride, bicarbonate, blood urea nitrogen, creatinine, glucose), PT, PTT
- Consider NG lavage, erythromycin 1–3 mg/kg or metoclopramide 10 mg IV to improve visualization
- Consider ICU admission for patients with significant comorbidities, hemodynamic instability, or high risk of rebleeding, and intubation for patients at high risk for aspiration
- Start high-dose proton pump inhibitors—omeprazole 40 mg orally twice a day, or omeprazole 80 mg IV bolus, then 8 mg/hr continuous IV infusion
- In patients with possible cirrhosis or portal hypertension, start octreotide 50 µg IV bolus, then 50–100 µg/hr continuous IV infusion

Upper endoscopy within 24 hours

Ulcer hemorrhage—continue proton pump inhibitor therapy

Variceal hemorrhage—see Figure 8-2

Unsuccessful endoscopic therapy

Successful endoscopic therapy

Repeat upper endoscopy

Two unsuccessful attempts at endoscopic therapy

Consider another upper endoscopy vs. surgery or angiography

Successful therapy

Prevention of rebleeding:
- Test and treat for *H. pylori*, and confirm eradication
- Discontinue NSAIDs, aspirin; if aspirin or NSAIDs are medically necessary, give them in conjunction with proton-pump inhibitors when acute bleeding episode resolves
- Acid suppression—omeprazole 20–40 mg orally daily

FIGURE 8–1. Algorithm for acute GI bleeding. CBC = complete blood count, PT = prothrombin time, PTT = activated partial thromboplastin time, NG = nasogastric, ICU = intensive care unit. Rockey DC. Gastrointestinal Bleeding. In: Feldman M, Friedman LS, and Sleisenger MH, editors. *Sleisenger and Fordtran's Gastrointestinal and Liver Disease,* 7th ed. Philadelphia. WB Saunders; 2002. p. 216. Adapted with permission, 2005.

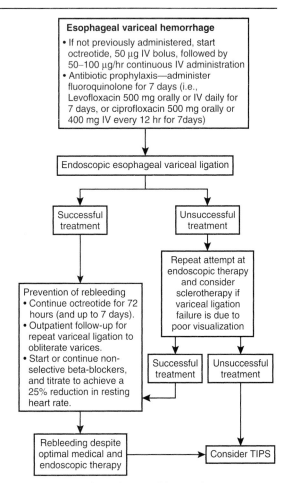

FIGURE 8–2. Esophageal variceal hemorrhage treatment. TIPS = transjugular intrahepatic portosystemic shunt. Rockey DC. Gastrointestinal Bleeding. In: Feldman M, Friedman LS, and Sleisenger MH, editors. *Sleisenger and Fordtran's Gastrointestinal and Liver Disease,* 7th ed. Philadelphia. WB Saunders; 2002. p. 216. Adapted with permission, 2005.

- ○ Platelet count should be kept above 50,000/μL.
- Basic metabolic panel should be obtained. A BUN: Creatinine ratio greater than 20 suggests the possibility of an upper GI source (although this may also be seen in a patient with a "pre-renal" cause of acute renal failure).
- Prothrombin time (PT) and activated partial thromboplastin time (PTT): Presence of any coagulopathy should be corrected.
  - ○ International Normalized Ratio (INR) > 1.5 should be corrected with fresh frozen plasma initially, and, if necessary (i.e., patients on Coumadin with supratherapeutic INR levels) Vitamin K_1, 10 mg given intravenously over 20 to 60 minutes.

EKG and cardiac enzymes should be obtained in patients with risk factors for coronary artery disease.

Nasogastric lavage with tap water should be performed in patients with upper GI bleeding.

High-dose proton pump inhibitors, such as omeprazole 40 mg orally twice a day, should be initiated. Intravenous administration may also be used (i.e., omeprazole 80 mg bolus, then 8 mg/hr for 72 hr). A neutral pH enhances clot formation and decreases clot breakdown.

Radiologic Imaging

Plain films of the abdomen may be obtained to rule out complications, such as perforation, but have little role in the diagnosis and management of upper gastrointestinal bleeding.

Barium studies may obscure visualization of a bleeding source during upper endoscopy and should not be performed.

Preparation for Endoscopy

Esophagogastroduodenoscopy (EGD) is the initial test of choice for acute upper GI bleeding. EGD is diagnostic in more than 95% of cases of upper GI bleeding and provides prognostic information as well.

Patients should be kept NPO, and a nasogastric (NG) lavage should be performed with warm tap water to clear the stomach of blood and blood clots. If the NG lavage is unsuccessful at clearing the stomach, 10 mg of metoclopramide or 1 to 3 mg/kg of erythromycin may be given intravenously prior to endoscopy to improve visualization.

Optimally, patients should be volume resuscitated and hemodynamically stabilized, with endoscopy performed within 24 hours of presentation. However, patients with persistent hypotension despite volume resuscitation, with ongoing hematemesis, hematochezia, or bloody NG lavage, and patients with cirrhosis should be evaluated with endoscopy sooner.

An INR less than 1.5 is required for endoscopic therapy. In patients with an INR greater than 1.5 who require emergent endoscopic intervention, the procedure may be performed with concurrent fresh frozen plasma infusion.

DEFINITIVE MANAGEMENT

Gastroduodenal Ulcer Bleeding

Background

Gastroduodenal ulcers account for up to 57% of upper GI bleeds. Risk factors for ulcer bleeding include NSAID use, age > 65, and a history of peptic ulcer disease.

NSAIDs and aspirin reduce production of protective prostaglandins, induce platelet dysfunction, and increase the risk of ulcer hemorrhage in a dose-dependent fashion. The relative risk of upper GI bleeding due to NSAID use ranges from 1.3 for COX-2 inhibitors to 7 for certain NSAIDs; aspirin has a relative risk of 1.6 to 2.8. The relative risk of upper GI bleeding for patients taking a COX-2 inhibitor, compared with a nonselective NSAID, ranges from 0.4 to 0.5.

Use of glucocorticoids with NSAIDs results in a 10-fold increase in the risk of upper GI bleeding compared to NSAID use alone. Ethanol intake also increases the risk of NSAID-induced ulcer bleeding. For example, ethanol use combined with aspirin at a dose of 325 mg daily results in a relative risk of upper GI bleeding of 7. Anticoagulant therapy and use of more than one NSAID also increases the risk of acute upper GI bleeding.

Although *H. pylori* infection is a risk factor for peptic ulcer disease, it remains unclear whether *H. pylori* is an independent risk factor for NSAID-induced acute upper GI bleeding.

Medical Therapy (Table 8-1)

Use of proton pump inhibitors following successful endoscopic intervention has been shown to decrease rebleeding rates, transfusion requirements, and need for surgical intervention. Proton pump inhibitors should be given at dosages equivalent to omeprazole 40 mg orally twice a day, or 80 mg IV bolus, followed by 8 mg/hr. Therapy at these dosages should be continued for 3 to 4 days.

Although H2 blockers may be useful in decreasing long-term rebleeding rates during maintenance therapy, their effectiveness in decreasing short-term rebleeding rates or transfusion requirements has been disappointing. This is likely due to their inability to maintain adequate acid suppression.

A meta-analysis that examined the efficacy of octreotide in nonvariceal bleeding demonstrated a 47% reduced risk of continued bleeding or rebleeding. This effect was greater for ulcer bleeding than for non-ulcer bleeding (52% vs 38% risk reduction).

In summary, high-dose proton pump inhibitors are the cornerstones of medical therapy for gastroduodenal ulcer hemorrhage. They reduce

Table 8-1. Medical Therapy for Acute GI Bleeding	
Ulcer Hemorrhage	
Intervention	**Outcome**
H2 blockers	Maintenance therapy reduces long-term rebleeding rates
	No effect on short-term transfusion requirements or rebleeding rates
H. pylori eradication	Likely decreased rebleeding rates at 1 year
Proton pump inhibitors	When given following successful endoscopic intervention, results in:
	Reduced transfusion requirements, rebleeding rates, repeat endoscopies, and need for surgical therapy
	No effect on mortality if given without endoscopic therapy
	Omeprazole 40 mg orally twice a day, or omeprazole 80 mg IV bolus, then 8 mg/hr (or equivalent dose of another proton pump inhibitor) should be administered following endoscopy

the risk of rebleeding when used in conjunction with endoscopic therapy.

Procedural Therapy

Endoscopic stigmata of bleeding gastroduodenal ulcers have significant prognostic value (Table 8-2). Clean, white-based ulcers and ulcers with a flat

Table 8-1. Medical Therapy for Acute GI Bleeding

Variceal Hemorrhage	
Intervention	**Outcome**
Nonselective beta-blockers	Decreases risk of initial hemorrhage
	Reduces mortality from variceal hemorrhage
	No effect on overall mortality
	Decreases risk of recurrent variceal hemorrhage
Octreotide	Decreases failure rate of initial hemostatic therapy
	Decreases transfusion requirements
	No mortality benefit
Antibiotic prophylaxis during acute variceal hemorrhage	Decreases risk of spontaneous bacterial peritonitis
	Improves survival in patients with variceal hemorrhage

Table 8-2. Endoscopic Stigmata of Gastroduodenal Ulcer Hemorrhage

	Rebleeding Rate	
Finding	**Without Endoscopic Therapy**	**With Endoscopic Therapy**
Arterial bleeding	85%–90%	20%
Active bleeding	55%	20%
Visible vessel	43%–50%	15%
Adherent clot	22%–40%	<5%
Oozing	10%–27%	<10%
Flat spot	5%–10%	<1%
Clean ulcer base	<3%	N/A

pigmented spot have less than 10% risk of rebleeding, even without endoscopic therapy. Ulcers with active arterial spurting or bleeding, visible vessel, or adherent clot are at high risk of rebleeding with medical therapy alone. Thus, endoscopic therapy is directed at high-risk ulcers.

The cornerstones of endoscopic therapy for bleeding gastroduodenal ulcers are epinephrine injection, thermal coagulation, or a combination of the two. Mechanical hemostasis with hemo-clips may also be used. For ulcers with active arterial bleeding, combination therapy is usually used. Adherent clots are usually removed and the underlying ulcers are subsequently treated with combination therapy. Visible vessels and oozing ulcers are treated with monotherapy only. Ulcers with flat pigmented spots or a clean white base are not treated endoscopically.

Despite advances in endoscopic therapy for ulcer hemorrhage, rebleeding occurs in up to 25% of cases. If rebleeding occurs, another attempt at endoscopic treatment is warranted. Despite lower rates of hemostasis, repeat endo-scopic therapy is associated with lower rates of complications.

Angiography should be considered in patients who fail repeated endoscopic treat-ments, or are poor operative candidates. Surgery should be reserved for patients who fail multiple attempts at endoscopic hemostasis.

Prevention of Rebleeding

Prevention of recurrent ulcer hemorrhage involves:

- Discontinuation of NSAID use
- *H. pylori* eradication
- Acid suppression

NSAIDs and aspirin should be discontinued in patients with NSAID-induced ulcer hemor-rhage. If this is not medically feasible, the following two strategies may be used:

- Proton pump inhibitors (PPIs) should be administered in conjunction with the NSAID or aspirin. Omeprazole 20–40 mg orally daily (or equivalent dose of a different PPI) may be used. PPIs and misoprostol 800 µg daily have equivalent ulcer healing rates, but PPIs have higher long-term remission rates. PPIs significantly lower the rebleeding rates in patients with a history of ulcer hemorrhage.
- Tests for *H. pylori* should be obtained, and *H. pylori* should be eradicated if present. During an acute upper GI bleed, endoscopy-based tests, such as the CLO (Campylobacter-like organism) test, may be falsely negative. Therefore, *H. pylori* serologies or a urease breath test should be used.

H. pylori should be eradicated in patients with acute ulcer hemorrhage, because eradication leads to a 3% to 33% reduction in rebleeding rates. *H. pylori* eradication should be confirmed with a urease breath test 6 weeks after cessation of therapy.

Acid suppression should be maintained with PPI therapy. See Box 8-3 for a summary of rebleeding prevention therapy in patients with ulcer hemorrhage.

Gastroesophageal Variceal Bleeding

Background

Gastroesophageal varices are present in up to 60% of patients with end-stage liver disease. Variceal bleeding has a mortality rate of 30% to 50% per event, and accounts for up to one third of deaths in patients with end-stage liver disease. Between 25% and 40% of patients with esophageal varices will have significant hemorrhage each year. Variceal bleeding tends to occur in the early morning and late evening hours, and has a 60% to 70% risk of rebleeding in the first 24

Box 8-3. Prevention of Recurrent Bleeding in Patients with Ulcer Hemorrhage and Esophageal Variceal Bleeding

Ulcer Hemorrhage

- Proton pump inhibitor therapy for acid suppression at a dose equivalent of omeprazole 20–40 mg orally daily
- Cessation of NSAID or aspirin use
- Assess for *Helicobacter pylori* infection, and eradicate if present

    During an acute upper GI bleed, endoscopy-based CLO testing may be falsely negative; histological evaluation, urease breath testing, or serologic testing may be better

- If NSAIDs or aspirin must be continued:

    Administer omeprazole 20–40 mg orally daily

    Assess for *H. pylori* infection, and eradicate if present

Esophageal Variceal Bleeding

- Titrate non-selective beta-blocker to decrease resting heart rate by 25%
- Obliterate varices with esophageal variceal ligation
- Encourage alcohol cessation in patients with alcoholic cirrhosis
- TIPS placement in patients with recurrent variceal bleeding despite optimal medical and endoscopic therapy

---

hours. Patients with gastric varices, encephalopathy, alcoholic cirrhosis, and large or actively bleeding varices have a higher risk of rebleeding. A portal pressure gradient greater than 12 mm Hg is associated with an increased risk of variceal bleeding.

Gastric varices may occur in 20% of patients with portal hypertension, and are usually found in conjunction with esophageal varices. Patients with isolated gastric fundic varices should be evaluated for splenic vein thrombosis (usually due to a pancreatic process). Gastric varices may be classified as:

- Type I—gastric varices that extend caudally from esophageal varices
- Type II—gastric fundic varices that are continuous with esophageal varices
- Type III—isolated gastric fundic varices

The size of the varices, underlying liver disease (as measured by Child-Turcotte-Pugh Class), and presence of stigmata of recent hemorrhage determine the risk for variceal bleeding. Prognosis correlates with underlying liver function; patients with the most severe liver disease have the worst prognosis.

Primary Prophylaxis

Nonselective beta-blockers, such as propanolol and nadolol, are used for primary prophylaxis in patients with esophageal varices. These medications reduce the risk of initial bleeding from 25% to 15%, and reduce mortality from variceal hemorrhage, but do not significantly decrease overall mortality. The dose of medication should be titrated to achieve a 25% reduction in the resting heart rate.

The use of nitrates in conjunction with beta-blockers results in a greater decrease in portal pressures, but has not been shown to decrease mortality. Esophageal variceal ligation, sclerotherapy, and transjugular intrahepatic portosystemic shunts should not be used routinely for primary prophylaxis of variceal hemorrhage.

Therapy for Acute Variceal Hemorrhage

Initial management for acute variceal hemorrhage involves obtaining intravenous access, fluid resuscitation, correction of coagulopathies, and transfusions if necessary. The hematocrit should be maintained at 30%. Higher levels may raise portal pressures and increase the risk of rebleeding.

Patients presenting with acute upper GI bleeding that have history, physical examination, or laboratory findings suspicious for cirrhosis should be started on octreotide (a somatostatin analogue) for presumed variceal hemorrhage. Octreotide is given as a 50-μg bolus, followed by 50 to 100 μg/hr continuous IV infusion. The use of octreotide is associated with lower transfusion requirements and increases the success rate of initial hemostasis; however, it has no effect on mortality. Octreotide should be continued for 3 to 7 days after endoscopic therapy for esophageal variceal hemorrhage.

Other agents used to treat variceal bleeding include vasopressin (with nitroglycerine) and terlipressin. Somatostatin has a significantly lower complication rate than vasopressin, but their hemostasis failure rates are comparable. Comparison of octreotide with terlipressin showed no difference in hemostasis or mortality. However, terlipressin is not available for use in the United States.

Variceal hemorrhage is also associated with an increased risk of infections, particularly spontaneous bacterial peritonitis. Thus, 7 days of prophylactic antibiotic therapy should be initiated with a fluoroquinolone, such as ciprofloxacin 400 mg IV or 500 mg orally every 12 hours for 7 days.

Sclerotherapy and esophageal variceal ligation are the two endoscopic modalities used to treat variceal bleeding. Although both are effective, band ligation is preferred to sclerotherapy because it eliminates esophageal varices in fewer sessions, results in a lower risk of rebleeding, and has a lower complication rate. Patients should be kept on a clear liquid diet for 24 hours after variceal ligation therapy. Band ligation should not be used for gastric varices; sclerotherapy is the endoscopic treatment of choice for gastric varices.

Esophageal variceal ligation and sclerotherapy have a 90% success rate in achieving hemostasis in variceal bleeding. In patients who rebleed, repeat endoscopic therapy should be performed. However, approximately 10% of patients with variceal hemorrhage will fail two attempts at endoscopic hemostasis. Placement of a transjugular intrahepatic portosystemic shunt (TIPS) should be considered in these patients. TIPS has a 90% success rate for hemostasis, with a goal of achieving a portal pressure gradient less than 12 mmHg. TIPS should be used cautiously in patients with advanced liver disease, hepatic encephalopathy, or impaired renal function, and is absolutely contraindicated in patients with right heart failure, primary pulmonary hypertension, polycystic liver disease, portal vein thrombosis with cavernous transformation, and severe liver disease. Long-term complications of TIPS include hepatic encephalopathy and worsening liver function. A Doppler ultrasound to assess TIPS patency should be performed the day after placement and every 3 months thereafter.

Prevention of Rebleeding

Obliteration of esophageal varices with repeat endoscopic variceal ligation should be used in conjunction with administration of nonselective beta-blockers (propanolol or nadolol), titrated to reduce resting heart rate by 25%. Combination medical and endoscopic therapy appears to have a lower rebleeding rate, and possibly a lower mortality rate, than endoscopic therapy alone.

Patients who rebleed despite adequate medical and endoscopic treatment should be considered for TIPS placement.

REFERENCES

Textbook Chapters

1. Rockey DC. Gastrointestinal Bleeding. In: Feldman M, Friedman LS, and Sleisenger MH,

editors. *Sleisenger and Fordtran's Gastrointestinal and Liver Disease,* 7th ed. Philadelphia. WB Saunders; 2002. pp. 211–226.

2. Bass NM, Yao FY. Portal Hypertension and Variceal Bleeding. In: Feldman M, Friedman LS, and Sleisenger MH, editors. *Sleisenger and Fordtran's Gastrointestinal and Liver Disease,* 7th ed. Philadelphia. WB Saunders; 2002. pp. 1487–1515.

Practice Guidelines

1. Eisen GM, Baron TH, Dominitz JA, et al. American Society for Gastrointestinal Endoscopy. Standards of Practice Committee. The role of endoscopic therapy in the management of variceal hemorrhage. *Gastrointes Endosc.* 2002;56:618–620.

2. Eisen GM, Dominitz JA, Faigel DO, et al. American Society for Gastrointestinal Endoscopy. Standards of Practice Committee. An annotated algorithmic approach to upper gastrointestinal bleeding. *Gastrointes Endosc.* 2001;53:853–858.

3. American Society for Gastrointestinal Endoscopy. The role of endoscopy in the management of non-variceal acute upper gastrointestinal bleeding. *Gastrointes Endosc.* 1992;38:760–764.

Review Article

Sharara AI, Rockey DC. Gastroesophageal variceal hemorrhage. *N Engl J Med.* 2001; 345:669–681.

General

Wolfe MM, Lichtenstein DR, Singh G. Gastrointestinal toxicity of nonsteroidal anti-inflammatory drugs. *N Engl J Med.* 1999; 340:1888–1899.

Therapy

1. Lin HJ, Lo WC, Lee FY, et al. A prospective randomized comparative trial showing that omeprazole prevents rebleeding in patients with bleeding peptic ulcer after successful endoscopic therapy. *Arch Int Med*. 1998; 158:54–58.

2. Khuroo MS, Yattoo GN, Javid G, et al. A comparison of omeprazole and placebo for bleeding peptic ulcer. *N Engl J Med*. 1997;336:1054–1058.

3. Lau JY, Sung JJ, Lee KK, et al. Effect of intravenous omeprazole on recurrent bleeding after endoscopic treatment of bleeding peptic ulcers. *N Engl J Med*. 2000;343:310–316.

4. Lau JY, Sung JJ, Lam YH, et al. Endoscopic retreatment compared with surgery in patients with recurrent bleeding after initial endoscopic control of bleeding ulcers. *N Engl J Med*. 1999;340:751–756.

5. Corley DA, Cello JP, Adkisson W, et al. Octreotide for acute esophageal variceal bleeding: A meta-analysis. *Gastroenterology* 2001;120:946–954.

6. Gotzsche PC. Somatostatin analogues for acute bleeding esophageal varicies. *Coch Data System Rev*. 2002;(1)CD000193.

7. Steigmann GV, Goff JS, Michaletz OP, et al. Endoscopic sclerotherapy as compared with endoscopic ligation for bleeding esophageal varicies. *N Engl J Med*. 1992; 326:1527–1532.

8. Gimson AE, Ramage JK, Panos MZ, et al. Randomized trial of variceal banding ligation versus injection sclerotherapy for bleeding esophageal varicies. *Lancet* 1993; 342:391–394.

9. Banares R, Albillos A, Rincon D, et al. Endoscopic treatment versus endoscopic plus pharmacologic treatment for acute variceal bleeding: A meta-analysis. *Hepatology* 2002;35:609–615.

References
Box 8-2

1. Rockey DC. Gastrointestinal Bleeding. In: Feldman M, Friedman LS, and Sleisenger MH, editors. *Sleisenger and Fordtran's Gastrointestinal and Liver Disease,* 7th ed. Philadelphia. WB Saunders; 2002. p. 214.
2. Eisen GM, Dominitz JA, Faigel DO, et al. American Society for Gastrointestinal Endoscopy. Standards of Practice Committee. An annotated algorithmic approach to upper gastrointestinal bleeding. *Gastrointes Endosc.* 2001;53:853–858.
3. Chang EB. Gastrointestinal Bleeding. In: *Digestive Diseases Self-Education Program* IV. Dubuque: Kendall/Hunt; 2004. p. 113.

Table 8-2

1. Eisen GM, Baron TH, Dominitz JA, et al. American Society for Gastrointestinal Endoscopy. Standards of Practice Committee. The role of endoscopic therapy in the management of variceal hemorrhage. *Gastrointes Endosc.* 2002;56:618–620.
2. Chang EB. Gastrointestinal Bleeding. In: *Digestive Diseases Self-Education Program IV.* 2004. pp. 116–117.
3. Laine L, Peterson WL. Bleeding peptic ulcer. *N Engl J Med.* 1994;331:717–727.
4. Rockey DC. Gastrointestinal Bleeding. In: Feldman M, Friedman LS, and Sleisenger MH, editors. *Sleisenger and Fordtran's Gastrointestinal and Liver Disease,* 7th ed. Philadelphia. WB Saunders; 2002. p. 219.

Hematology

Anemia

KEY POINTS

1. Anemia refers to reduced red blood cell (RBC) mass.

2. The mean corpuscular volume represents the average RBC size and is used to classify the type of anemia as microcytic, normocytic, or macrocytic.

3. Microcytic anemia results from processes that impair hemoglobin synthesis in the RBC, such as iron deficiency, lead poisoning, sideroblastic anemia, and thalassemia.

4. Some causes of normocytic anemia include chronic renal failure, anemia of chronic disease, hypogonadism, aplastic anemia, myelodysplastic syndrome, and bone marrow infiltration.

5. Causes of macrocytic anemia include DNA synthesis defects (folate deficiency, vitamin B_{12} deficiency, myelodysplastic syndrome, nucleotide analogs) hypothyroidism, liver disease, and alcoholism.

6. The reticulocyte count differentiates a hypoproliferative anemia (such as iron, folate, or B_{12} deficiency) from a hyperproliferative anemia (such as hemolysis or acute blood loss).

7. Patients with anemia may be asymptomatic (especially if the anemia is mild or develops slowly) or may have symptoms of fatigue, lightheadedness, exercise intolerance, dyspnea, or worsening angina.

8. Initial testing should include a complete blood count with differential, reticulo-

cyte count, and stool guaiac. Other useful tests include (a) lactate dehydrogenase, haptoglobin, and total and direct bilirubin if hemolysis is suspected, (b) ferritin, serum iron, and total iron binding capacity (TIBC) if the anemia is microcytic, and (c) vitamin B_{12} and folate if the anemia is macrocytic.

9. When iron deficiency anemia is diagnosed, a search for the cause of the deficiency is mandatory.

10. Anemia of chronic disease can usually be distinguished from iron deficiency on the basis of the ferritin, serum iron concentrations, and TIBC.

11. Neurological disease (which can occur in the absence of anemia) is a potential complication of vitamin B_{12} deficiency but not of folate deficiency.

12. Definitive diagnosis of vitamin B_{12} deficiency in patients with low vitamin B_{12} levels that are above the lower limit of the normal range requires measurement of methylmalonic acid and homocysteine.

13. Nonfasting serum folate concentrations < 2 ng/mL are diagnostic of folate deficiency whereas levels > 4 ng/mL essentially rule out folate deficiency.

14. Hemolytic anemia develops when the bone marrow cannot compensate for a shortened RBC lifespan. Findings supporting a diagnosis of hemolysis include reticulocytosis, splenomegaly, fragmented RBCs on the peripheral smear ("helmet cells," or schistocytes), increased serum lactate dehydrogenase, unconjugated hyperbilirubinemia (unconjugated bilirubin comprising 80% of the total bilirubin), and reduced haptoglobin concentrations.

DEFINITIONS

Anemia: Reduced red blood cell (RBC) mass.

Hemoglobin concentration (Hgb): Grams of hemoglobin per 100 mL of whole blood (g/dL).

Red blood cell (RBC) count: Number of RBCs (in millions) per microliter of whole blood.

Mean corpuscular volume (MCV): Average RBC size. The MCV is commonly used to classify anemia as "microcytic" (RBCs smaller than normal), "normocytic" (normal-sized RBCs), or "macrocytic" (RBCs larger than normal), which provides a framework for determining the cause of the anemia (Box 9-1). Since the MCV is an average measure of RBC size, the MCV may be normal if microcytic and macrocytic cells are simultaneously present (for example, concurrent iron and vitamin B_{12} deficiency). As a general rule of thumb, normal RBCs are approximately the size of a lymphocyte nucleus on the peripheral blood smear.

Hematocrit: Percent of whole blood volume occupied by RBCs. The hematocrit is calculated using the RBC count and MCV as follows:

$$\text{Hematocrit}\,(\%) = \text{MCV}\,(\text{femtoliters})$$
$$\times \text{RBC count}\,(\times 10^6/\mu l) \times 10$$

The normal value for the hematocrit depends on age, gender, and possibly race. The World Health Organization defines anemia as hematocrit < 39% in adult men and < 36% in adult women. Hemoglobin concentration, hematocrit, and RBC count are calculated using RBC mass and blood volume. Therefore, low blood volumes in patients with dehydration or acute blood loss may mask anemia that will become evident following volume repletion.

Box 9-1. Common Causes of Anemia

Microcytic

Iron deficiency

Anemia of chronic disease (typically normocytic)

Thalassemia

Sideroblastic anemia

Lead poisoning

Normocytic

Subacute blood loss

Anemia of chronic disease

Bone marrow abnormality

Hemolysis

Sickle cell disease

Renal insufficiency

Macrocytic

Reticulocytosis

Vitamin B_{12} deficiency

  Pernicious anemia

  Intestinal disease (gastrectomy, ileal disease or resection, blind intestinal loops, bacterial overgrowth)

  Nutritional deficiency (vegans)

  Diphyllobothrium latum (fish tapeworm)

Folate deficiency

  Intestinal malabsorption (Crohn's, celiac disease)

  Nutritional deficiency ("tea and toast" elderly diet, alcoholism)

  Drug-induced (methotrexate, trimethoprim, phenytoin, alcohol, oral contraceptives)

  Liver disease

  Hypothyroidism

  Alcoholism

  Hereditary spherocytosis

  Drugs (methotrexate, zidovudine, hydroxyurea, trimethoprim)

Adapted from Hematology/Oncology. In: Ferri FF, editor. *Practical Guide to the Care of the Medical Patient*, 6th ed. St. Louis: Mosby; 2004.

Mean corpuscular hemoglobin (MCH): Amount of hemoglobin (in picograms) per RBC and is calculated by:

$$\frac{\text{Hgb(g/dl)}}{\text{RBC count}\,(\times 10^6/\mu l)} \times 10$$

Mean corpuscular hemoglobin concentration (MCHC): Hemoglobin concentration (gm/dL) per RBC (i.e., the amount of hemoglobin per RBC relative to the RBC size) and is calculated by:

$$\frac{\text{Hgb (g/dl)}}{\text{Hematocrit (\%)}} \times 100 \quad \text{OR} \quad \frac{1}{\text{MCV}} \times \text{MCH}$$

Red cell distribution width (RDW): A measure of the variation in RBC size (expressed as a percentage). The greater the variation, the greater the RDW. The RDW provides useful information when used together with the MCV. For example, a patient with concurrent microcytic and macrocytic anemia may have a normal MCV but the RDW should be elevated (because there is variability in cell size).

Reticulocyte count: The reticulocyte is the precursor of the mature RBC and is formed when the nucleus is extruded from a normoblast. The reticulocyte retains its ribosomal machinery for approximately 4 days, of which 3 days are usually spent in the bone marrow. Reticulocytes spend 1 day in the peripheral blood, representing approximately 1% of total circulating RBCs. On a standard blood smear with Wright Giemsa stain, reticulocytes are the bluish cells without central pallor that are larger than mature RBCs.

The reticulocyte count facilitates the workup of anemia by differentiating a hypoproliferative (for example, iron, folate, or vitamin B_{12} deficiency) from a hyperproliferative anemia (for example, hemolysis). The reticulocyte count should be corrected for the degree of anemia and the change in reticulocyte maturation time. This adjusted measure is known as the reticulocyte production index (RPI) and is calculated as follows:

$$RPI = \frac{\text{Reticulocyte count (\%)} \times \dfrac{\text{Patient's hematocrit}}{45\%}}{\text{Maturation Factor}}$$

Hematocrit (%)	Maturation Factor
45	1.0
35	1.5
25	2.0

In response to anemia, reticulocytes move from the bone marrow to the peripheral blood sooner. Therefore, reticulocytes can spend upwards of 2 days in the circulation. However, the increased numbers of circulating reticulocytes in this setting does not represent increased RBC production rates. Therefore, we recommend using the maturation factor so that the longer reticulocyte circulating times do not overestimate the reticulocyte response.

A low RPI (< 2) suggests a hypoproliferative anemia (i.e., impaired RBC production in response to the anemia). Typical causes of a low RPI include iron, folate, or vitamin B_{12} deficiency, or bone marrow injury, failure, or infiltration (Box 9-2). A high RPI (> 3) suggests a hyperproliferative anemia (i.e., increased RBC production in response to anemia), as occurs with hemolysis, acute blood loss, and recovery of the bone marrow from infection or nutrient deficiency.

SIGNS AND SYMPTOMS OF ANEMIA

Signs and symptoms are less likely if the anemia develops slowly or is mild. Patients may be asymptomatic or complain of fatigue, lightheadedness, exercise intolerance, dyspnea, or worsening angina.

Box 9-2. The Reticulocyte Production Index (RPI)

RPI < 2 (Hypoproliferative Anemia)

Iron deficiency

Folate deficiency

Vitamin B_{12} deficiency

Bone marrow dysfunction (aplastic anemia, myelodysplasia)

Bone marrow infiltration (leukemia)

Bone marrow injury (cancer chemotherapy, radiation therapy)

Reduced erythropoietin (chronic renal failure)

Hypothyroidism

Hypogonadism

RPI > 3 (Hyperproliferative Anemia)

Hemolysis

Bone marrow response to acute blood loss

Bone marrow recovery from infection or nutrient deficiency

Physical exam may reveal pallor of the conjunctivae, nail beds, palmar creases, or face. Cardiovascular exam may reveal a systolic ejection murmur (increased aortic flow caused by increased cardiac output) and bounding peripheral pulses. Acute blood loss may present with signs of hypovolemia, such as hypotension. The etiology of the anemia may be suggested by the presence of specific history or physical examination clues, such as pica (appetite for substances inappropriate to eat, such as clay or dirt, sometimes seen with iron deficiency), smooth, beefy red tongue (vitamin B_{12} deficiency), lymphadenopathy (cancer), scleral icterus (hemolysis), petechiae or ecchymoses (thrombocytopenia), melena, hematochezia, hematemesis, or menorrhagia (blood loss).

Laboratory Data (Table 9-1)

Initial testing should include:

- Complete blood count with differential and examination of a blood smear
- Reticulocyte count

Table 9-1. Sensitivity and Specificity of Tests Used in the Diagnosis of Anemia		
	Sensitivity (%)	Specificity (%)
Iron Deficiency Anemia		
Ferritin		
< 15 ng/mL	59	99
< 30 ng/mL	92	98
< 41 ng/mL	98	98
Pernicious anemia		
Anti-parietal cell antibodies	> 90	50
Anti-intrinsic factor antibodies	50–84	98
Vitamin B_{12} Deficiency		
Increased homocysteine AND methylmalonic acid	94	99
Folate Deficiency		
Increased homocysteine AND normal methylmalonic acid	86	99
Hemolysis		
Serum haptoglobin ≤ 25 mg/dL	83	96
↑ lactate dehydrogenase AND ↓ haptoglobin		90

- Stool guaiac
- Lactate dehydrogenase, haptoglobin, and bilirubin (total and direct) if hemolysis is suspected
- Ferritin, serum iron, and total iron-binding capacity (TIBC) if the patient has normocytic anemia with increased RDW or microcytic anemia
- Vitamin B_{12} and folate, if the patient has a normocytic anemia with increased RDW or macrocytic anemia
- Hematology consultation for bone marrow biopsy if the anemia is associated with pancytopenia or there are abnormal cells in the peripheral circulation

Microcytic (MCV < 80 fL) Anemia

Microcytic anemia usually results from processes that impair hemoglobin synthesis in the RBC such as iron deficiency (Fig. 9-1), anemia of chronic disease (reduced iron availability), lead poisoning or sideroblastic anemia (reduced heme synthesis), or thalassemias (reduced globin production).

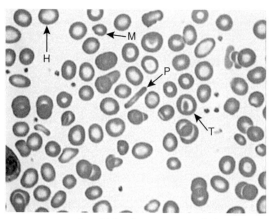

FIGURE 9–1. Peripheral blood smear—iron deficiency anemia. H=hypochromic red cell; P=pencil cell; T=target cell; M=microcytic cell. Reproduced with permission from Provan D, Weatherall D. Red cells II: Acquired anemias and polycythemia. *Lancet* 2000;355:1260–1268.

1. Iron Deficiency Anemia

Iron deficiency is the most common cause of anemia. In humans, iron is absorbed by duodenal cells, transported in plasma by transferrin, and stored in the body mostly as ferritin. When iron deficiency develops, serum iron and ferritin concentrations decline. Because ferritin is an acute phase reactant, levels may be normal or elevated in patients with a concurrent inflammatory condition. Iron deficiency stimulates transferrin gene expression. Therefore, transferrin concentrations (also measured as total iron-binding capacity, or TIBC) are increased in patients with iron deficiency. As a result, the transferrin saturation, defined as the ratio of serum iron to TIBC will be low (typically, < 10%).

When iron deficiency anemia is diagnosed, a search for the cause of the deficiency is indicated. Initially, a colonoscopy and esophagogastroduodenoscopy may be performed. If these tests are negative, evaluation of the small intestines may be required. Common causes include menstrual or gastrointestinal blood loss; malabsorption (for example, celiac sprue) is less common.

Treatment of Iron Deficiency

Iron is best absorbed in a mildly acidic gastric environment. Therefore, iron tablets should not be taken within 2 hours of antacids. Ascorbic acid (vitamin C) 250 mg or a glass of orange juice or grapefruit juice with each iron tablet will improve absorption. We recommend starting with ferrous sulfate, because it is cheap and well absorbed. The optimal dose of ferrous sulfate is 325 mg three times daily (between meals). To improve tolerability, we recommend starting with 325 mg once daily and titrating slowly to goal. We also recommend a stool softener to prevent constipation. Patients who are intolerant of this dosing regimen (nausea, constipation, abdominal cramping) can try taking the iron less frequently (for example, twice a day). If side effects persist, another iron formulation, such as polysaccharide-iron complex, can be tried. Iron supplementation should be continued until the anemia has resolved although some experts continue treatment for up to 6 months longer to completely replenish iron stores.

Patients who fail to respond to iron supplementation may be noncompliant, may not be absorbing the iron (malabsorption syndrome, taking iron with antacids or acid-blocking medications), may have blood loss that exceeds the ability to replace iron orally, may have a coexisting illness interfering with the response, or may have another cause for the microcytic anemia.

2. Thalassemia

α-thalassemia and β-thalassemia result from a reduction or absence of the α-globin and β-globin chains of hemoglobin, respectively. The thalassemias are typically found in patients originating from Africa, the Mediterranean, Middle East, Southeast Asia, and the Indian subcontinent. Thalassemias have a broad spectrum of presentation, depending on the severity of the globin chain defect. Patients with severe forms of this disorder are diagnosed in childhood. In adults, a diagnosis of thalassemia is usually considered when patients originating from one of the regions of the world mentioned previously are incidentally found to have a hypochromic, microcytic anemia but no evidence of iron deficiency. The diagnosis of β-thalassemia is suggested by the presence of a low MCV and MCH but normal RDW and can be confirmed with hemoglobin electrophoresis. There is no simple test for diagnosing mild forms of α-thalassemia. This diagnosis is likely in patients belonging to high prevalence populations who have microcytosis and a normal RDW but minimal or no anemia and no evidence of iron deficiency or β-thalassemia. Mild forms of the thalassemias require no medical therapy although genetic counseling may be appropriate.

3. Anemia of Chronic Disease

Anemia of chronic disease is immune-mediated and occurs in patients with chronic infections, inflammatory conditions, cancer, and systemic disorders. This anemia is characterized by multiple abnormalities including a reduced RBC lifespan, an abnormal response to erythropoietin, and increased uptake and retention of iron by reticuloendothelial cells. The diversion of iron from the circulation into storage sites results in limited availability of iron for new RBC formation. Anemia of chronic disease causes a microcytic or normocytic anemia and can be distinguished from iron deficiency on the basis of the ferritin, serum iron concentrations, and total iron-binding capacity (Table 9-2). When the two conditions coexist, diagnosis of iron deficiency can be difficult because these three test parameters are altered. In this case, measurement of the soluble transferrin receptor concentration (which should be upregulated in patients with iron deficiency but normal in patients with anemia of chronic disease), a judicious trial of iron supplementation, or bone-marrow aspirate may be useful.

Table 9-2. Differentiating Iron Deficiency Anemia and the Anemia of Chronic Disease

	Serum Iron	TIBC	Iron/ TIBC	Ferritin
Iron deficiency anemia	↓	↑	↓	↓
Anemia of chronic disease	↓	↓ or →	↓	↑ or →
Both	↓	↓	↓	↓ or →
Thalassemia	↑	↓	↑	↑

From Weiss G, Goodnough LT. Anemia of chronic disease. *N Engl J Med.* 2005;352:1011–1023.
TIBC = total iron binding capacity, Iron/TIBC = transferrin saturation, Both = co-existing iron deficiency anemia and anemia of chronic disease.

Normocytic (MCV 80–100 fL) Anemia

Normocytic anemia has a wide range of causes, including chronic renal failure (reduced erythropoietin production), anemia of chronic disease, early iron deficiency anemia, endocrine disease (anterior pituitary dysfunction, hypogonadism, thyroid deficiency or excess), aplastic anemia (from drugs, viruses, or idiopathic; reticulocytes should be absent), myelodysplastic syndrome, and marrow replacement by tumor cells.

Macrocytic (MCV > 100 fL) Anemia

Causes of macrocytic anemia include reticulocytosis (reticulocytes are larger than normal RBCs), folate or vitamin B_{12} deficiency (required for nucleic acid synthesis in RBC precursors), medications including zidovudine or hydroxyurea (anti-metabolites that interfere with nucleic acid synthesis), abnormal RBC maturation (myelodysplastic syndrome), hypothyroidism, liver disease, and alcoholism.

1. Vitamin B_{12} Deficiency

Vitamin B_{12} (cobalamin) is required for DNA synthesis. Strict vegans may develop vitamin B_{12} deficiency because animal products (meat, eggs, milk) are the best dietary source of this vitamin. Deficiency of vitamin B_{12} causes macrocytic anemia (unless there is coexisting iron-deficiency anemia, thalassemia, or anemia of chronic disease) because the resulting defect in DNA synthesis impairs cell division whereas RNA synthesis and the synthesis of cytoplasmic components remain unaffected. Vitamin B_{12} deficiency can also cause neurological symptoms such as paresthesias, loss of vibratory sense, and if severe, subacute combined degeneration of the spinal cord (posterior and lateral column lesions that are specific for vitamin B_{12} deficiency and result from defective myelin formation), and dementia. Posterior column signs include

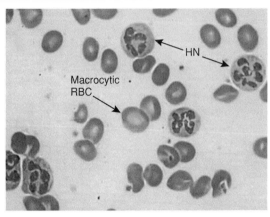

FIGURE 9–2. Peripheral blood smear—megaloblastic anemia. HN=hypersegmented neutrophil; RBC=red blood cell. Reproduced with permission from Provan D, Weatherall D. Red cells II: Acquired anemias and polycythemia. *Lancet* 2000;355:1260–1268.

sensory ataxia with a positive Romberg's sign and loss of vibration and position sense. Lateral column signs include spasticity, limb weakness, and a positive Babinski sign. These neurological symptoms can occur in the absence of anemia.

With vitamin B_{12} deficiency, the peripheral smear may show thrombocytopenia, leukopenia, hypersegmented neutrophils (at least one neutrophil with 6 or more lobes), and macrocytosis (Fig. 9-2). Lactate dehydrogenase and serum bilirubin levels may be high because there is ineffective erythropoiesis and early RBC destruction (this is also true for folate deficiency; see following text).

The diagnosis of vitamin B_{12} deficiency is straightforward when levels of this vitamin are low. Falsely low vitamin B_{12} levels have been reported in pregnant patients, women using oral contraceptives, and in patients who are folate deficient. Subtle deficiencies characterized by low vitamin B_{12} levels that are still above the lower limit of the normal range require further testing for confirmation—measurement of methylmalonic acid and homocysteine. Both are elevated in patients with vitamin B_{12} deficiency, but only homocysteine is elevated in patients with folate deficiency (Fig. 9-3).

Pernicious Anemia

Vitamin B_{12} absorption in the terminal ileum requires intrinsic factor, which is produced by gastric parietal cells. The most common cause of vitamin B_{12} deficiency is pernicious anemia, which refers to autoimmune gastric atrophy leading to impaired production of intrinsic factor.

Pernicious anemia increases the risk for gastric carcinoma and gastric carcinoid and has been associated with other autoimmune disorders including Hashimoto's thyroiditis, type 1 diabetes mellitus, Addison's disease, vitiligo, and primary ovarian failure.

The presence of anti-parietal cell antibodies is very sensitive but not specific for pernicious anemia (see Table 9-1). In contrast, anti-intrinsic factor antibodies are very specific but not sensitive for pernicious anemia. The Schilling test is not routinely performed nowadays. This test demonstrates low urinary excretion of orally administered vitamin B_{12} that improves when intrinsic factor is co-administered.

For treatment of vitamin B_{12} deficiency, we recommend intramuscular vitamin B_{12} 1000 μg (1 mg) daily for one week, then 1000 μg weekly for one month, then 1000 μg monthly for life if the cause of the vitamin B_{12} deficiency cannot be corrected (for example, pernicious anemia). These doses are safe and inexpensive. Neurologic abnormalities may resolve over months if treatment is not delayed. Alternatively, a daily dose of 1000 to 2000 μg orally can be used even in patients with pernicious anemia or a poorly functioning terminal ileum, because 1% of vitamin B_{12} is absorbed by mass action even in the absence of intrinsic factor. This approach

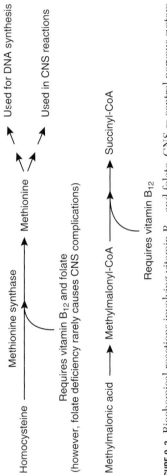

FIGURE 9–3. Biochemical reactions involving vitamin B_{12} and folate. CNS = central nervous system.

requires strict patient compliance, which should be monitored with recommend periodic measurements of vitamin B_{12} levels.

During the early treatment of severe vitamin B_{12} deficiency, patients can develop significant hypokalemia because potassium is required for new hematopoietic cell production.

2. Folate Deficiency

Folate is also required for DNA synthesis. Therefore, folate deficiency also leads to macrocytic anemia and hypersegmented neutrophils. The elderly eating a "tea and toast" diet are at risk for folate deficiency because dietary sources of folate include vegetables, fruits, cereals, and dairy products. Body stores of folate are considerably less than those for vitamin B_{12}; therefore, folate deficiency can develop within months of malabsorption or reduced intake. Measurement of serum folate concentrations is the initial screening test for folate deficiency. Nonfasting levels < 2 ng/mL are diagnostic of folate deficiency in the absence of anorexia. Levels > 4 ng/mL essentially rule out folate deficiency, although one hospital meal can normalize serum folate levels in patients who are folate deficient. In this setting or when folate values are intermediate (2–4 ng/mL), it is appropriate to measure RBC folate levels. This test is expensive and should not be used for screening.

The recommended treatment for folate deficiency is 1 mg folic acid daily for several months. Longer treatment is appropriate if the underlying cause for the anemia cannot be corrected (for example, malabsorption). Folic acid can partially correct the megaloblastic anemia of vitamin B_{12} deficiency but will have no effect on the neurologic manifestations. Therefore, every patient with megaloblastic anemia should be tested for vitamin B_{12} deficiency, even if folate deficiency has been confirmed.

Hemolytic Anemia (Box 9-3)

Hemolytic anemia develops when the bone marrow is unable to compensate for a shortened RBC lifespan. If the patient presents for the first time in adult life, the hemolysis is likely acquired, and the cause is almost always of extracorpuscular (i.e., arising from outside the RBC) origin. Examples include injury to RBCs as they transverse prosthetic heart valves, antibodies directed against RBCs, and hypersplenism.

Hemolysis can be classified as immune or nonimmune and intravascular (immediate lysis

Box 9-3. Classification of the Hemolytic Anemias with Examples

Intravascular Hemolysis

Intravenous infusion of hypotonic solution

ABO blood type incompatibility transfusion reaction

Microangiopathy (such as prosthetic heart valve injury to red blood cells)

Extravascular Hemolysis

  Extracorpuscular

   Hypersplenism

   Autoimmune hemolytic anemia (warm or cold auto-antibodies)

   Drug-induced

  Intracorpuscular

   Sickle cell disease and other hemoglobinopathies

   Hereditary spherocytosis and other membrane defects

   Glucose-6-phosphate dehydrogenase deficiency and other enzyme deficiencies occurring in the circulation due to severe RBC damage) or extravascular (RBC destruction in the reticuloendothelial system—spleen, bone marrow, lymph nodes, and liver). Immune hemolytic anemia may be autoimmune (antibodies directed against self-RBCs), allo-immune (for example, hemolytic transfusion reactions), or drug-induced (penicillin, quinidine, quinine). Autoimmune hemolytic anemia is classified as "warm" if the antibodies (IgG) bind RBCs most strongly at body temperature and "cold" if the antibodies (usually IgM) bind RBCs most strongly at 0° to 4°C. Therefore, patients with cold autoimmune hemolytic anemia have symptoms related to cold exposure. Lymphoproliferative disorders, infections, and some medications can cause warm hemolytic anemia, although most cases are idiopathic. Some causes of cold hemolytic anemia include *Mycoplasma pneumoniae*, infectious mononucleosis, and lymphoproliferative disorders.

Findings supporting a diagnosis of hemolysis include reticulocytosis (which attempts to compensate for the shortened RBC survival times), splenomegaly, fragmented RBCs on the peripheral smear ("helmet cells" or schistocytes), increased serum lactate dehydrogenase (enzyme released from hemolyzed RBCs), unconjugated hyperbilirubinemia (excess bilirubin from rapid hemoglobin degradation overwhelms the liver's ability to conjugate), and reduced haptoglobin concentrations (haptoglobin binds free hemoglobin and the complex is rapidly cleared by the liver). We recommend consultation with a hematologist for further evaluation and management when hemolysis is suspected or confirmed.

REFERENCES

Review Articles

1. Provan D, Weatherall D. Red cells I: Inherited anaemias. *Lancet* 2000;355:1169–1175.

2. Provan D, Weatherall D. Red cells II: Acquired anaemias and polycythaemia. *Lancet* 2000;355:1260–1268.
3. Spivak JL. The blood in systemic disorders. *Lancet* 2000;355:1707–1712.

Specific Disorders

1. Andres E, Loukili NH, Noel E, et al. Vitamin B_{12} (cobalamin) deficiency in elderly patients. *CMAJ* 2004;171:251–259.
2. Andrews NC. Disorders of iron metabolism. *N Engl J Med*. 1999;341:1986–1995.
3. Gehrs BC, Friedberg RC. Autoimmune hemolytic anemia. *Am J Hematol*. 2002; 69:258–271.
4. Olivieri NF. The β-thalassemias. *N Engl J Med*. 1999;341:99–109.
5. Toh BH, van Driel IR, Gleeson PA. Pernicious anemia. *N Engl J Med*. 1997;337:1441–1448.
6. Weiss G, Goodnough LT. Anemia of chronic disease. *N Engl J Med*. 2005;352:1011–1023.

Diagnosis

1. Snow CF. Laboratory diagnosis of vitamin B_{12} and folate deficiency: A guide for the primary care physician. *Arch Intern Med*. 1999; 159:1289–1298.
2. Bain BJ. Diagnosis from the blood smear. *N Engl J Med*. 2005;353:498–507.

Venous Thromboembolism

KEY POINTS

1. Venous thromboembolism (VTE) refers to deep vein thrombosis (DVT) and pulmonary embolism (PE).
2. The risk of PE from proximal (above-the-calf) lower-extremity DVT is ~50%.
3. Up to 50% of patients with first-time VTE have no obvious risk factors for VTE.
4. Acquired risk factors for VTE include surgery, medical illness (such as cancer, myocardial infarction, heart failure, and stroke), oral contraceptives, hormone replacement therapy, antiphospholipid antibodies, and hyperhomocysteinemia.
5. Inherited risk factors for VTE include factor V Leiden, the prothrombin gene mutation, antithrombin III deficiency, and protein C and S deficiencies.
6. Signs and symptoms of lower-extremity DVT include edema, erythema, warmth, and pain of the involved limb.
7. Signs and symptoms of PE include dyspnea, tachypnea, tachycardia, cough, hemoptysis, pleuritic chest pain, syncope, and cyanosis.
8. Compression ultrasonography is the recommended first-line test for patients with suspected DVT (sensitivity 97%–100%, specificity 98%–99% for proximal DVT).
9. Chest CT is the recommended initial imaging test for inpatients with suspected PE. Third-generation CT scanners reliably rule PE in or out.

First-generation CT scanners may miss a small (< 5 mm) PE.

10. Screening for thrombophilia is controversial. These tests have the highest yield when patients present with recurrent, idiopathic VTE, a family history of VTE, or a history of recurrent, unexplained pregnancy loss.

11. Intravenous unfractionated heparin (UFH) is used as a "bridge" to warfarin for treatment of VTE. There are "fixed-dose" and "weight-based" algorithms for adjusting heparin doses to achieve a therapeutic effect.

12. Subcutaneous low molecular weight heparin is an alternative to UFH that achieves predictable levels of anticoagulation without the need for laboratory monitoring of anti-factor Xa levels (unless the patient is obese or has renal failure).

13. Warfarin should only be initiated when therapeutic levels of heparin have been achieved. A typical starting dose is 5 mg daily with a goal International Normalized Ratio (INR) of 2.0 to 3.0.

14. Factors influencing the duration of anticoagulation (3 months to indefinite) include (a) the patient's risk of bleeding, (b) whether the VTE is idiopathic or associated with a major temporary risk factor, (c) whether the VTE is a first-time or recurrent event, and (d) whether there is a high risk for recurrence.

15. Thrombolysis is sometimes used for extensive or limb-threatening DVT but carries a higher risk of hemorrhage than standard anticoagulation.

16. Mechanical prophylaxis against VTE is appropriate for low-risk patients and those with a contraindication to anticoagulation. Pharmacologic prophylaxis is

recommended for medical or surgical patients at moderate to high risk for VTE.

17. Inferior vena cava (IVC) filters reduce the risk of short-term PE from proximal DVT but increase the risk of recurrent DVT and do not reduce mortality. Indications include (a) proximal DVT with a contra-indication to anticoagulation and (b) recurrent PE despite therapeutic anticoagulation.

EPIDEMIOLOGY

Venous thromboembolism (VTE) refers to deep vein thrombosis (DVT) and pulmonary embolism (PE). In the general population, VTE occurs in 1 per 1000 persons each year in the United States, although the frequency increases with advancing age. The risk of PE from proximal (above-the-calf) lower extremity DVT is approximately 50%, and the mortality rate from PE exceeds 15% in the first 3 months following diagnosis.

PATHOPHYSIOLOGY

Virchow's triad (venous stasis, vessel wall injury, and hypercoagulability) summarizes the mechanisms by which acquired and inherited risk factors (Table 10-1) predispose to VTE. Typically, lower-extremity thrombus develops in valve pockets of the calf veins. Although most of these thrombi lyse spontaneously, approximately one fourth of untreated calf vein thrombi extend into the proximal veins. Thrombus that sufficiently impairs venous return through the affected vein will lead to increased venous and capillary pressures and subsequently edema. Massive thrombosis can compromise venous outflow from the leg (phlegmasia cerulean dolens).

Table 10-1. Acquired and Inherited Risk Factors for Venous Thromboembolism

Acquired Risk Factors	Inherited Risk Factors
Age	Antithrombin III
Antiphospholipid	deficiency
antibodies	Factor V Leiden
Cancer	Protein C deficiency
Central venous	Protein S deficiency
catheter	Prothrombin gene
Chronic care facility	mutation
resident	
Critical illness	
Heparin-induced	
thrombocytopenia	
Hormone replacement	
therapy	
Hyperhomocysteinemia*	
Hypertension	
Immobilization	
Long-haul flights	
Medical illness (e.g., CHF,	
COPD)	
Obesity	
Oral contraceptives	
Pregnancy	
Stroke with extremity	
paresis	
Surgery	
Thoracic outlet syndrome	
Tobacco use	
Trauma	
Varicose veins	

Adapted from Gelfand EV, et al. *Venous Thromboembolism Guidebook*, 4th ed. *Crit Path Cardiol*. 2003;2:247–265.
CHF, congestive heart failure; COPD, chronic obstructive pulmonary disease.
*Hyperhomocysteinemia can be inherited (rare).

PE most commonly originates from veins of the pelvis and lower extremities. PE of sufficient size can increase right ventricular afterload, which may lead to right ventricular dilatation, tricuspid regurgitation, and right heart failure.

Mechanisms of hypoxemia from PE include ventilation–perfusion mismatch, atelectasis (resulting from loss of surfactant and alveolar hemorrhage), and shunting (venous blood not passing through ventilated gas exchange units of the lung before returning to the arterial circulation). In acute PE, intracardiac shunting can occur through a patent foramen ovale when right atrial pressure exceeds left atrial pressure.

RISK FACTORS

The known major risk factors for VTE are summarized in the following text. Up to one half of patients who present with first-time VTE have no readily identifiable risk factors.

Surgery

Patients at high risk for post-operative VTE are over 40 years of age; undergoing surgery for cancer, neurosurgery, major vascular surgery, or orthopedic leg surgery lasting more than 30 minutes; or have a personal history of VTE or additional risk factors for VTE. DVT is usually diagnosed during the third to sixth postoperative days, but the risk for thrombosis persists for several months.

Cancer

Virtually any cancer can present with DVT, but typical sites of malignancy include the pancreas, ovary, liver, and brain. Idiopathic VTE probably increases the risk of a subsequent diagnosis of cancer, especially within the first year following the thrombotic event. The benefit of extensively searching for cancer in patients with primary VTE is uncertain and has not been shown to be cost-effective. Therefore, a complete medical history, physical examination, routine laboratory tests, chest x-ray, age-appropriate cancer screening are all that is currently recommended for these patients.

Medical Illness

Other medical illnesses associated with VTE include myocardial infarction, chronic obstructive pulmonary disease, heart failure, hypertension, nephrotic syndrome, stroke, and polycythemia vera. The highest incidence of VTE in critically ill patients not receiving prophylaxis occurs in acute spinal cord patients. More frequent use of central venous catheters for dialysis, parenteral nutrition, and chemotherapy has increased the incidence of upper extremity DVT, which has been reported in up to one-fourth of patients with these catheters.

Oral Contraceptives and Hormone Replacement Therapy

Hormone replacement therapy (HRT), raloxifene (selective estrogen receptor modulator), and oral contraceptives are risk factors for VTE. Oral contraceptives and HRT substantially increase the risk of VTE in women with a coexisting thrombophilia, such as Factor V Leiden. However, routine screening for thrombophilia is not recommended prior to initiating these medications because the absolute risk for VTE in these patients is low. A history of VTE is an absolute contraindication to exogenous estrogen use.

Antiphospholipid Antibodies

Antiphospholipid antibodies may occur as a primary thrombotic or obstetrical disorder known as the antiphospholipid antibody syndrome or can be seen in association with other medical disorders, such as systemic lupus erythematosus. Antiphospholipid antibodies predispose to arterial and venous thrombosis and recurrent pregnancy loss. A definitive diagnosis of the antiphospholipid antibody syndrome requires the presence of clinical criteria (such as recurrent, spontaneous abortions and arterial or venous thrombosis) in the setting of persistent laboratory abnormalities (lupus anticoagulant antibodies or moderate-to-high levels of IgG or IgM anticardiolipin antibodies detected on two occasions at least 6 weeks apart).

Hyperhomocysteinemia

Hyperhomocysteinemia, typically defined as fasting homocysteine levels greater than 15 μmol/L (greater than the 95th percentile of the general population), is a risk factor for arterial and venous thrombosis. The mechanism of thrombosis is unknown. Hyperhomocysteinemia is most commonly caused by folate deficiency exacerbated by vitamin B_{12} or vitamin B_6 deficiencies. Other causes of hyperhomocysteinemia include genetic defects in the methylenetetrahydrofolate reductase and methionine synthase enzymes, folate antagonists (such as methotrexate and phenytoin), and renal insufficiency (homocysteine is metabolized predominantly by the kidneys). Regardless of etiology, most patients with hyperhomocysteinemia respond to multivitamin treatment. Folic acid is the most effective therapy and will reduce homocysteine levels even when patients are not obviously folate deficient. Clinical trials are currently underway to determine whether these therapies ultimately reduce the frequency of subsequent thrombosis.

Factor V Leiden

Factor V Leiden refers to an abnormal factor V protein resulting from a point mutation in the factor V gene. This mutation, which is most prevalent in people of northern European descent, renders the protein relatively resistant to degradation by the endogenous anticoagulant, protein C. As a result, factor V remains active, increases thrombin generation, and predisposes to VTE. Factor V Leiden increases the risk for a first episode of VTE and is the most common known inherited cause of VTE. There is conflicting data as to whether patients with Factor V Leiden have an increased risk of recurrent VTE.

Prothrombin Gene Mutation

The prothrombin gene mutation is the second most common genetic abnormality predisposing to VTE. Prothrombin (factor II) is a precursor of thrombin. A point mutation in an untranslated region of the prothrombin gene results in higher plasma prothrombin levels and increases the risk for a first episode of VTE.

Antithrombin III Deficiency

Antithrombin III (ATIII) is a naturally occurring anticoagulant that limits thrombosis by inactivating procoagulant factors. ATIII deficiency can be acquired (e.g., in cirrhosis), but only the inherited form appears to carry a risk for initial and recurrent VTE. The risk of VTE in surgical patients with ATIII deficiency is extremely high, in part, because surgery further reduces ATIII levels. Heparin and acute VTE lower ATIII levels; therefore, ATIII deficiency cannot be diagnosed in these settings.

Protein C and Protein S Deficiencies

Protein C is a naturally occurring anticoagulant that requires protein S as a cofactor for its reactions. More than 100 mutations in the protein C or protein S genes have been detected that reduce protein level or function and predispose to VTE. Protein C and S deficiencies are rare causes of VTE. Warfarin inhibits the synthesis of all vitamin K–dependent proteins, including protein C and S; therefore, protein C or S deficiency cannot be diagnosed during concurrent warfarin use.

SIGNS AND SYMPTOMS OF VENOUS THROMBOEMBOLISM

Patients with lower-extremity DVT may present with edema, erythema, warmth, and pain of the involved limb. Occasionally, a palpable cord and prominent superficial collateral veins may be present. Physical examination may reveal a low-grade fever or a positive Homan's sign (this test refers to calf pain with dorsiflexion of the foot but has poor sensitivity for DVT).

Dyspnea is the most frequent symptom of PE and tachypnea is the most common sign of PE. A small PE that causes infarction near the pleura is more likely to present with cough, hemoptysis, and pleuritic chest pain. Massive PE can present with dyspnea, syncope, and cyanosis. Other signs of PE include tachycardia, jugular venous distension, and accentuation of the pulmonic component of the second heart sound.

The differential diagnosis for PE and DVT is summarized in Table 10-2. PE can be a diagnostic challenge. Young patients with excellent cardiac reserve may present with subtle symptoms whereas PE in older patients may masquerade as other diseases, such as an acute coronary syndrome or exacerbation of chronic obstructive pulmonary disease.

LABORATORY DATA

Initial laboratory testing for patients with VTE should include the following (obtaining some of these tests may depend upon the clinical situation):

1. Baseline complete blood count, creatinine, international normalized ratio (INR), and activated partial thromboplastin time (aPTT).

Table 10-2. Differential Diagnosis for Deep Vein Thrombosis and Pulmonary Embolism

Deep Vein Thrombosis	Pulmonary Embolism
Cellulitis	Acute coronary syndrome
Extrinsic compression of iliac vein	Acute exacerbation of chronic obstructive pulmonary disease
Lymphangitis	Anemia
Lymphedema	Anxiety
Peripheral edema	Aortic dissection
Post-thrombotic syndrome	Asthma
Ruptured Baker's cyst	Bronchitis
Ruptured tendon or muscle	Musculoskeletal pain
Superficial thrombophlebitis	Pericardial tamponade
Venous insufficiency	Pneumonia
	Pneumothorax
	Pulmonary edema
	Pulmonary hypertension
	Rib fracture

Adapted from Gelfand EV, et al. *Venous Thromboembolism Guidebook*, 4th ed. *Crit Path Cardiol*. 2003;2:247–265.

2. **D-Dimer** is produced when endogenous fibrinolysis causes plasmin to digest some of the fibrin clot that is part of the thrombus. Therefore, D-dimer is elevated in almost all patients with VTE. However, an elevated D-dimer cannot be used to diagnose VTE because this test is abnormal in many other conditions, including inflammation, surgery, and cancer. However, a normal D-dimer in an outpatient or emergency room patient with a low clinical probability of VTE safely excludes DVT and PE. D-Dimer testing is not recommended for hospitalized patients because this test will be elevated in most inpatients. If PE is suspected in a hospitalized patient, chest CT is recommended as the first-line diagnostic test (see following text).

3. **Electrocardiogram (ECG)** is useful for excluding unrelated cardiac causes of the

patient's symptoms, such as acute myocardial infarction and acute pericarditis. If the PE causes right ventricular strain, the ECG may show T wave inversion in leads V_1 through V_4 and new right bundle branch block. If the PE is sufficiently large, the ECG will show the classic S1Q3T3 pattern (S wave in lead I, a Q wave in lead III, and an inverted T wave in lead III). A normal ECG is very unusual in patients with acute PE.

4. **Chest x-ray** is useful for excluding other causes for the patient's symptoms, such as pneumonia, pneumothorax, rib fracture, and heart failure. Sometimes, there are findings on chest x-ray suggestive of PE, such as cardiomegaly, pulmonary artery enlargement, and Hampton's Hump (wedge-shaped density at the periphery of the lung, occasionally seen with small PE).

5. **Hypercoagulable workup** see "When to Test for Hypercoagulable States" (p. 202). Protein C and S deficiencies cannot be diagnosed while the patient is receiving warfarin. Antithrombin III deficiency cannot be diagnosed while the patient is receiving heparin or is in the immediate postoperative setting.

6. **Echocardiogram** is not usually required unless the patient is acutely ill and there is a need to exclude non-PE causes for the patient's symptoms, such as acute myocardial infarction, pericardial tamponade, and aortic dissection.

The arterial blood gas is not useful for diagnosing PE. Hypoxemia has poor specificity for PE and the partial pressure of oxygen on room air and the alveolar–arterial oxygen gradient are normal in approximately 20% of PE patients.

Troponins are sometimes slightly elevated in patients with PE, presumably because of strain and micro-infarction of the right ventricle, not atherosclerosis.

IMAGING TESTS

Compression Ultrasonography

Ultrasonography is the recommended first-line test for patients with suspected DVT. Thrombus is diagnosed when there is failure of the vein to fully collapse when pressure is applied with the ultrasound probe. Absence of blood flow with color Doppler is also used to detect thrombus. Compared with venography, ultrasonography has a sensitivity of 97% to 100% and a specificity of 98% to 99% for proximal DVT but is less accurate for diagnosing calf vein thrombosis (sensitivity approximately 50% to 70% and positive predictive value 80%).

Contrast Venography

Contrast venography is the "gold-standard" diagnostic test for DVT but is invasive and has potential contraindications. Therefore, this test is reserved for patients with high clinical probability for VTE despite normal ultrasound studies or patients with equivocal ultrasound results.

Chest CT

Chest CT has become the first-line imaging test for diagnosing PE. To interpret the CT results accurately, the generation of the CT scanner must be known. First-generation scanners have 5 mm resolution and may fail to detect smaller PEs. If your institution has first-generation scanners only, lower-extremity ultrasonography is a reasonable option if the chest CT is negative. However, absence of lower-extremity DVT does not exclude PE because the thrombus may have completely embolized to the lung (if suspicion for PE persists, the patient should undergo pulmonary angiography. Third-generation scanners have 1 mm resolution and can more reliably rule out PE.

Chest CT also offers other advantages—thrombus can be directly visualized and alternative diagnoses that are not evident on chest x-ray, such as pneumonia or interstitial fibrosis, may be identified.

Ventilation–Perfusion Lung Scan

The ventilation–perfusion lung scan has been traditionally used to evaluate suspected PE. Lung scans are useful if they are normal or show a high probability for PE but most scans are nondiagnostic (intermediate or indeterminate). Therefore, this test is now becoming a second-line diagnostic test for PE and is used when patients cannot undergo chest CT scanning (e.g., renal insufficiency or history of allergy to the contrast agent). A chest x-ray is needed to properly interpret the ventilation–perfusion lung scan.

Pulmonary Angiogram

Pulmonary angiography is the gold standard diagnostic test for PE but is rarely used nowadays. The complication rate from this procedure is low when performed by experts. Pulmonary angiography is occasionally used when there is high clinical suspicion for PE but lung imaging and lower extremity ultrasonography studies are normal or nondiagnostic.

Diagnostic Algorithms

1. Deep vein thrombosis

For outpatients, DVT can be safely excluded when the pre-test probability (based on medical history and physical examination) is low and the D-dimer is normal. Outpatients with a higher pre-test probability or an elevated D-dimer should undergo compression ultrasonography. Outpatients with a low pre-test probability for DVT who have an elevated D-dimer and normal ultrasonography testing should undergo repeat ultrasonography one week later to fully exclude DVT.

Inpatients with suspected DVT should undergo compression ultrasonography without measurement of D-dimer (D-dimer is elevated in many hospitalized patients without VTE).

2. Pulmonary embolism

Wells criteria can be used to rapidly assess the likelihood of PE at the bedside. A score of 4.0 or lower makes PE unlikely (PE risk < 5%). The seven features are (1) clinical signs and symptoms of DVT (3.0 points), (2) an alternative diagnosis is less likely than PE (3.0 points), (3) heart rate > 100 bpm (1.5 points), (4) immobilization or surgery in the preceding four weeks (1.5 points), (5) prior VTE (1.5 points), (6) hemoptysis (1.0 point), and (7) cancer treated currently or within the previous 6 months or palliative (1.0 point).

PE is virtually excluded in outpatients or emergency room patients with a normal D-dimer. Chest CT is the recommended initial imaging test if the D-dimer is elevated or the patient is hospitalized. The third-generation CT scanners reliably rule PE in or out. Patients with normal first-generation scanner images should undergo lower extremity ultrasonography. If the ultrasound exam is normal but there is high suspicion for PE, pulmonary angiography should be performed.

WHEN TO TEST FOR HYPERCOAGULABLE STATES

Screening for thrombophilia is controversial, because there is no clear evidence that there is improvement in outcome when treatment is modified because of a hypercoagulable state. These tests have the highest yield when patients present with recurrent, idiopathic VTE, a family history of VTE, or a history of recurrent, unexplained pregnancy loss. One approach is to test for factor V Leiden, the prothrombin gene mutation, hyperhomocysteinemia, and antiphospholipid antibodies, because the presence of these conditions may alter medical management. For example, the antiphospholipid antibody syndrome is treated with more intensive, prolonged anticoagulation than are other causes of VTE. Hyperhomocysteinemia is easily corrected with folate administration. Factor V Leiden is the most prevalent inherited thrombophilia and synergistically increases the risk of VTE in patients with the prothrombin gene mutation, hyperhomocysteinemia, or concurrent oral contraceptive use. We do not recommend routine testing for protein C or S deficiencies or antithrombin III deficiency because these abnormalities are rare.

TREATMENT

Absolute contraindications to anticoagulation include active bleeding, platelet count $\leq 20,000/mm$, and neurosurgery, ocular surgery, or intracranial hemorrhage within the past 10 days. Relative contraindications to anticoagulation include brain metastasis, recent major trauma, major abdominal surgery within the prior 2 days, and severe hypertension (systolic blood pressure > 200 mm Hg or diastolic blood pressure > 120 mm Hg).

Unfractionated Heparin

Intravenous unfractionated heparin (UFH) has traditionally been used as a "bridge" to warfarin for the treatment of VTE. There are several "fixed-dose" and "weight-based" algorithms for adjusting heparin doses to achieve therapeutic effect. One proposed starting dose is a bolus of 80 U/kg followed by a continuous infusion of 18 U/kg/hr. The aPTT should be monitored every 4 to 6 hours after initiation of heparin or change in heparin dose. The aPTT need only be monitored daily if the patient is clinically stable and the aPTT is in the therapeutic range (usually defined as 60–80 sec). A sample protocol for adjusting heparin dosages based on a nontherapeutic aPTT is presented in Table 10-3.

If heparin causes bleeding, discontinuation of the heparin infusion is usually sufficient. If there is life-threatening bleeding from heparin, protamine sulfate 1 mg/100 U of heparin administered over the preceding 4 hours (maximum dose 50 mg) should be given as a slow intravenous infusion. Patients using NPH insulin can have a severe allergic reaction to protamine.

Table 10-3. Example of a Weight-Based Nomogram for Achieving Therapeutic Heparin Levels

Variable	Heparin Dose
Initial heparin dose	80 U/kg bolus, then 18 U/kg/hr
aPTT < 35 sec	80 U/kg bolus, then increase infusion by 4 U/kg/hr
aPTT 35–59 sec	40 U/kg bolus, then increase infusion by 2 U/kg/hr
aPTT 60–89 sec	No change
aPTT 90–100 sec	Decrease infusion by 3 U/kg/hr
aPTT > 100 sec	Hold infusion for 1 hour, then decrease rate by 4 U/kg/hr

Adapted with permission from Raschke RA, Reilly BM, Guidry JR, Fontana JR, Srinivas S. The weight-based heparin dosing nomogram compared with a "standard care" nomogram. A randomized controlled trial. *Ann Intern Med.* 1993;119:874–881.

Low-Molecular-Weight Heparin

Low-molecular-weight heparin (LMWH) is derived from UFH and has a molecular weight of approximately 5000 daltons compared to 15,000 daltons for UFH. Whereas UFH inhibits both thrombin and factor Xa, LMWH preferentially has an anti-factor Xa effect. LMWH, administered as a subcutaneous injection, has revolutionized the treatment of DVT and offers several advantages over UFH as a bridge to warfarin. Patients with VTE and normal or near-normal renal function achieve predictable levels of anticoagulation with LMWH and can be treated as outpatients without laboratory monitoring. In contrast, patients receiving UFH often have wide fluctuations in anticoagulation intensity, especially during initial titration. LWMH is at least as effective and safe as UFH. In addition, LWMH causes less heparin-induced thrombocytopenia and osteoporosis than UFH and improves quality of life at lower cost.

Enoxaparin is an example of a LMWH that has been approved by the Food and Drug Administration for the:

1. Inpatient treatment of acute DVT with and without PE, dosed at 1 mg/kg twice daily or 1.5 mg/kg once daily
2. Outpatient treatment of acute DVT without PE, dosed at 1 mg/kg twice daily.

Outpatient treatment with LMWH is not appropriate for every patient with DVT. For example, patients presenting with large, extensive DVT are at risk for massive PE and should be hospitalized. LMWH is also not a good choice for the homeless, blind, or intravenous drug abusers. UFH, which has a much shorter half-life than LMWH, may be more desirable in surgical patients with VTE in whom rapid reversal of anticoagulation in the setting of bleeding may be necessary.

How to Monitor Low Molecular Weight Heparin Therapy

LMWH does not substantially raise the aPTT. Therefore, measurement of anti-Xa levels is used to assess the degree of anticoagulation with LMWH. The therapeutic range for anti-Xa levels 4 to 6 hours after the second or third dose of enoxaparin is 0.5 to 1.0 anti-Xa IU/mL. Since enoxaparin achieves a predictable level of anti-coagulation, routine measurement of anti-Xa levels is not indicated except in the setting of renal failure (LMWH is renally metabolized) or obesity (because of unpredictable absorption of LMWH).

Warfarin

Warfarin should only be initiated when thera-peutic levels of UFH or LMWH have been achieved. Therapeutic heparin levels will offset the temporary hypercoagulable state that occurs when warfarin depletes levels of proteins C and S (endogenous anticoagulants) before depleting the longer half-life procoagulant factors. Warfarin should be initiated at 5 mg daily (a smaller dose is reasonable in the elderly) with a goal INR of 2.0 to 3.0. The INR will not increase much during the first 48 hours of warfarin administration. Drug interactions (Table 10-4), malnourishment, and significant alcohol con-sumption may cause an exaggerated response to warfarin. Culprit drugs include amiodarone, acetaminophen, and some antibiotics, such as fluoroquinolones and sulfamethoxazole-tri-methoprim. An inappropriately low therapeutic response to warfarin occurs with rifampin, med-ication noncompliance, and diets rich in green leafy vegetables.

Heparin should be discontinued after a minimum of 5 days. One recommendation is to

Table 10-4. Major Drug Interactions with Warfarin

Anticoagulant Response Increased	Anticoagulant Response Decreased
Acetaminophen	Antithyroid drugs
Amiodarone	Barbiturates
17-alkyl androgens	Carbamazepine
Cimetidine	Cholestyramine
Clofibrate	Sucralfate
Disulfiram	
Erythromycin	
Fluconazole	
Fluoxetine	
Metronidazole	
High-dose salicylates	
Tamoxifen	
Trimethoprim-sulfamethoxazole	

From Schulman S. Care of patients receiving long-term anticoagulant therapy. *N Engl J Med.* 2003;349:675–683. Copyright © 2003 Massachusetts Medical Society. All rights reserved. Adapted with permission, 2005.

ensure that the INR is at least 2.3 when heparin is discontinued because heparin itself raises the INR slightly, and there is risk for developing a subtherapeutic INR if the INR is only 2.0 to 2.3 when the heparin is discontinued.

DURATION OF ANTICOAGULATION

Patients with a first-time DVT that developed in the setting of a major temporary risk factor, such as surgery or trauma, can be treated with anticoagulation for 3 months. Six months of anticoagulation is recommended for patients with first-time, idiopathic DVT. Patients at high risk for recurrence (for example, patients with lupus anticoagulant, antithrombin III deficiency, or recurrent VTE) often receive anticoagulation indefinitely. However, other factors such as patient preference and risk of bleeding enter into medical decision-making when determining the duration of anticoagulation. Low-intensity warfarin (target INR 1.5–2.0) after the patient has completed a full course of conventional anticoagulation for idiopathic DVT significantly reduces the risk of recurrent VTE and carries a low risk for bleeding. This approach may be a reasonable option for indefinite anticoagulation in some patients.

Patients with PE resulting from surgery or trauma can be treated with anticoagulation for 6 months. Almost all other patients with PE should receive anticoagulation indefinitely.

EXCESSIVE ANTICOAGULATION—WHAT TO DO?

If the INR is above 4.0 and there is no bleeding, warfarin can be withheld until the INR returns to the therapeutic range. Vitamin K can also be used to correct the INR but is inadequate if there is life-threatening bleeding (vitamin K takes 12 to 24 hours to reach full effect). Appropriate vitamin K dosages are 1 mg orally or 0.5 mg intravenously (subcutaneous injection has variable absorption). High vitamin K doses are not recommended because they can lead to warfarin resistance for several days. When the INR is very high or there is major bleeding, fresh frozen plasma (2–3 U initially) human recombinant factor VIIa concentrates, or prothrombin-complex concentrates can be used to avert or reverse bleeding safely and rapidly.

THROMBOLYTIC THERAPY

Thrombolysis is sometimes used in patients with extensive or limb-threatening DVT in an attempt to rapidly dissolve fresh thrombus and restore venous patency. Thrombolysis may reduce the risk of the post-thrombotic syndrome but carries a higher risk of hemorrhage than standard anticoagulation. Thrombolysis is also used in patients with massive PE (recombinant tissue plasminogen activator 100 mg over 2 hours without concomitant heparin). We recommend consultation with the hematology service when considering thrombolytic therapy.

PREVENTION OF VENOUS THROMBOEMBOLISM

Mechanical prophylaxis is appropriate for low-risk patients and patients with a contraindication to anticoagulation, and includes graduated compression stockings, intermittent pneumatic compression (stimulates endogenous fibrinolytic activity and also physically causes increased venous blood flow), and early ambulation in the postoperative period.

Pharmacologic prophylaxis is recommended for medical or surgical patients at moderate-to-high risk for VTE and includes subcutaneous UFH 5000 U two or three times daily or LMWH, such as subcutaneous enoxaparin 40 mg daily. These regimens do not increase the risk of bleeding.

Inferior vena cava (IVC) filters reduce the risk of short-term PE in patients with proximal DVT but increase the risk of recurrent DVT and do not reduce mortality. IVC filters are used in patients with proximal DVT who have a contraindication to anticoagulation or patients with recurrent PE despite therapeutic anticoagulation. Since IVC filters increase the risk of recurrent DVT, anticoagulation should be used concurrently when safe to do so.

POST-THROMBOTIC SYNDROME

Post-thrombotic syndrome occurs in one third of patients with proximal DVT (usually within 2 years of diagnosis) treated with anticoagulation (duration of anticoagulation has no effect on incidence) and is characterized by pain, swelling, and chronic skin changes. The incidence of this syndrome may be lower in patients treated with thrombolytic drugs or below-knee graduated elastic compression stockings (30–40 mmHg at the ankle). There is no way of identifying patients at risk for the post-thrombotic syndrome; therefore, all patients with DVT should be advised to wear compression stockings for the first 2 years following diagnosis.

REFERENCES

Review Articles

1. Kyrle PA, Eichinger S. Deep vein thrombosis. *Lancet* 2005;365:1163–1174.
2. Goldhaber SZ, Elliott CG. Acute pulmonary embolism part I: Epidemiology, pathophysiology, and diagnosis. *Circulation* 2003;108:2726–2729.
3. Goldhaber SZ, Elliott CG. Acute pulmonary embolism part II: Risk stratification, treatment, and prevention. *Circulation* 2003;108: 2834–2838.
4. Goldhaber SZ. Pulmonary embolism. *Lancet* 2004;363:1295–1305.
5. Joffe HV, Goldhaber SZ. Upper-extremity deep vein thrombosis. *Circulation* 2002;106:1874–1880.

Risk Factors

1. Seligsohn U, Lubetsky A. Genetic susceptibility to venous thrombosis. *N Engl J Med*. 2001;334:1222–1231.
2. Levine JS, Branch DW, Rauch J. The antiphospholipid syndrome. *N Engl J Med*. 2002;346:752–763.
3. Vandenbroucke JP, Rosing J, Bloemenkamp KWM, et al. Oral contraceptives and the risk

of venous thrombosis. *N Engl J Med*. 2001;
344:1527–1535.

Diagnosis

1. Schoepf UJ, Goldhaber SZ, Costello P. Spiral computed tomography for acute pulmonary embolism. *Circulation* 2004;109:2160–2167.
2. Kearon C, Hirsh J. The role of venous ultrasonography in the diagnosis of suspected deep venous thrombosis and pulmonary embolism. *Ann Intern Med*. 1998;129: 1044–1049.

Treatment

1. Weitz JI. Low-molecular-weight heparins. *N Engl J Med*. 1997;337:688–698.
2. Schulman S. Care of patients receiving long-term anticoagulant therapy. *N Engl J Med*. 2003;349:675–683.
3. Kucher N, Goldhaber SZ. Management of massive pulmonary embolism. *Circulation* 2005;112:e28–e32.
4. Bates SM, Ginsberg JS. Treatment of deep-vein thrombosis. *N Engl J Med*. 2004;351:268–277.

Prevention

1. Goldhaber SZ, Turpie AGG. Prevention of venous thromboembolism among hospitalized medical patients. *Circulation* 2005;111:e1–e3.
2. Goldhaber SZ. Prevention of recurrent idiopathic venous thromboembolism. *Circulation* 2004;110(Suppl IV), IV-20–IV-24.

SECTION V

Infectious Diseases

CHAPTER 11

Cellulitis and Diabetic Foot Infections

KEY POINTS

Cellulitis

1. Most cases of cellulitis are caused by gram-positive cocci (*Streptococcus pyogenes* and *Staphylococcus aureus*).
2. Patients with unusual exposures (see Table 11-1), recent antibiotic use, or vascular and lymphatic compromise may be at risk for infection by other organisms.
3. Blood and wound cultures should be reserved for patients with exposures listed in Table 11-1; lymphatic, vascular, or immune compromise; increased likelihood of resistant organisms; or lack of response to empiric therapy.
4. Patients with evidence of systemic toxicity or rapid progression of infection should receive inpatient parenteral therapy. Milder infections can be treated successfully in the outpatient setting.
5. Empiric therapy with nafcillin, dicloxacillin, or cefazolin should be initiated. Appropriate coverage for unusual exposures (see Table 11-1) should be given as well.

Diabetic Foot Infection

1. Neuropathy, vascular insufficiency, and hyperglycemia contribute to the development of foot ulcers, which subsequently become colonized and infected.

2. Acute infections are usually caused by gram-positive cocci.
3. Patients with chronic ulcers, recent hospitalizations, or recent antibiotic use may have a polymicrobial infection with gram-positive cocci, gram-negative bacteria, and resistant organisms.
4. Assessment of the patient with a diabetic foot infection should include the clinical status, any predisposing factors such as anatomic abnormalities or vascular insufficiency, the size and extent of the ulcer, and local complications such as abscess formation or osteomyelitis.
5. Biopsies of the cleaned and débrided wound site should be obtained.
6. Choice of empiric antibiotics depends on the infection severity and risk factors for resistant organisms.
7. Osteomyelitis should be suspected in patients with visible bone, bone that can be palpated using a metal probe, or ulcers that do not heal after 6 weeks of appropriate therapy.

DEFINITION AND EPIDEMIOLOGY

Cellulitis is a skin and subcutaneous tissue infection that can affect any part of the body. Cellulitis is most commonly caused by *Staphylococcus aureus* and *Streptococcus pyogenes*. However, other infectious agents may predominate in different clinical situations (Table 11-1). Although cellulitis is quite common, accurate incidence information is not available. Some estimates suggest that cellulitis accounts for approximately 2% of outpatient office visits, or up to 158 visits per 10,000 person-years.

The term *diabetic foot infection* refers to a spectrum of foot infections in patients with

Table 11-1. Probable Etiology of Soft Tissue Infections Associated with Some Specific Risk Factors or Settings

Risk Factor	Potential Infectious Organism	Treatment
Cat bite	*Pasteurella multocida*	Amoxicillin-clavulanate, ampicillin-sulbactam, cefoxitin. *P. multocida* is resistant to dicloxacillin and nafcillin
Dog bite	*P. multocida, Capnocytophaga canimorsus, Staphylococcus intermedius*	Amoxicillin-clavulanate, ampicillin-sulbactam, cefoxitin. *P. multocida* is resistant to dicloxacillin and nafcillin
Human bite	*Eikenella corrodens, Fusobacterium, Porphyromonas, Prevotella, S. pyogenes*	Amoxicillin-clavulanate, ampicillin-sulbactam, cefoxitin
Hot tub exposure	*Pseudomonas aeruginosa*	Aminoglycosides, third-generation cephalosporins, ticarcillin, mezlocillin, piperacillin, fluoroquinolones (in adults)
Diabetes mellitus or peripheral vascular disease	Group B streptococci	Penicillin or erythromycin
Periorbital cellulitis in children	*Haemophilus influenzae*	Third-generation cephalosporin

Table 11-1. Probable Etiology of Soft Tissue Infections Associated with Some Specific Risk Factors or Settings—cont'd

Risk Factor	Potential Infectious Organism	Treatment
Saphenous venectomy site	Groups C and G streptococci	Penicillin or erythromycin
Fresh water laceration	*Aeromonas hydrophilia*	Trimethoprim-sulfamethoxazole, fluoroquinolones, aminoglycosides, chloramphenicol, third-generation cephalosporins; resistant to ampicillin
Sea water exposure, raw oysters, and cirrhosis	*Vibrio vulnificus*	Tetracyclines
Stasis dermatitis or lymphedema	Groups A, C, G streptococci	Penicillin or erythromycin
Cat scratch, or bacillary angiomatosis in an HIV patient	*Bartonella henselae, B. quintana*	Erythromycin
Fish mongering, bone rendering	*Erysipelothrix rhusiopathiae*	Erythromycin, clindamycin, tetracycline, cephalosporins; resistant to sulfonamides, chloramphenicol

Fish tank exposure	*Mycobacterium marinum*	Rifampin and ethambutol
Contact with others with soft tissue infections	Methicillin-resistant *S. aureus*	Vancomycin
Compromised host with ecthyma gangrenosum	*P. aeruginosa*	Aminoglycosides, third-generation cephalosporins, ticarcillin, mezlocillin, piperacillin, fluoroquinolones (in adults)

Stevens DL. Cellulitis, pyoderma, abscesses and other skin and subcutaneous infections. In: Cohen J, Powderly WG, Berkley SF, et al. *Infectious Diseases*, 2nd ed. Philadelphia: Mosby; 2004. p. 133.

diabetes mellitus that ranges from a limited cutaneous infection to osteomyelitis, but most commonly refers to an infection of a foot ulcer. These foot infections are a major source of morbidity in patients with diabetes mellitus; more than one half of diabetics hospitalized with a foot infection subsequently require amputation.

Pathogenesis

Risk Factors for Cellulitis

General
Risk factors for cellulitis include obesity, vascular or lymphatic compromise (e.g., venous insufficiency, saphenous venectomy, or lymph node dissection after surgery for breast cancer), lower extremity edema, diabetes mellitus, and skin trauma (e.g., pressure ulcers, trauma or tinea pedis).

Patients without vascular or immune defects will likely be infected by *S. aureus* or group A streptococci. *Pseudomonas*, enterococci, or other bacteria may cause cellulitis in patients with an immune or vascular defect, or loss of significant skin integrity (e.g., burns).

Breast Cancer

Women who have undergone surgery for breast cancer with axillary lymph node dissection are at risk for recurrent cellulitis in the ipsilateral breast and upper extremity. Disruption of normal lymphatic drainage is thought to play a role in pathogenesis.

Saphenous Venectomy

Patients with saphenous venectomy are at increased risk for recurrent cellulitis because of vascular and perhaps lymphatic impairment. Tinea pedis appears to be a significant risk factor in this patient population, serving as a site of entry for microorganisms.

Pathogenesis of Cellulitis

Bacteria penetrate the cutaneous barrier through breaks in the skin or via hair follicles. Microbial cell wall components (e.g., endotoxins, peptidoglycans) stimulate production of chemo-tactic factors, which attract neutrophils to the region. Continued production of pro-inflamma-tory cytokines causes fever and local changes of erythema, edema, warmth, and pain.

Patients with decreased tissue perfusion as a result of vascular disease (e.g., atherosclerosis, diabetes) may have an increased susceptibility to cellulitis and are predisposed to deeper soft tissue infections.

Risk Factors for Diabetic Foot Infections

Diabetic foot infections occur as a result of multiple risk factors that result in an initial break in the protective skin barrier and an increased susceptibility to infection:

- Peripheral neuropathy
  - Motor neuropathy leads to changes in foot anatomy (neuro-osteoarthropathic deformities), resulting in deformities such as high arch and abnormal toe positioning that increase the risk of ulcer formation.
  - Sensory neuropathy decreases pain sensation so that diabetic patients are not aware of ulcer formation or injury.
  - Autonomic neuropathy causes dry skin that is more prone to trauma.
- Hyperglycemia negatively impacts wound healing and white blood cell (particularly polymorphonuclear cell) function.
- Peripheral vascular disease hinders wound healing, causes tissue ischemia, and impairs neutrophil chemotaxis.

Pathogenesis and Microbiology of Diabetic Foot Infections

The initial break in overlying skin is usually caused by trauma or pressure ulceration. The area becomes colonized with bacteria, and becomes infected over a period of hours to days.

- Acute infection in an antibiotic-naïve patient who has not been recently hospitalized is usually caused by gram-positive cocci (*S. aureus* and beta-hemolytic streptococci).
- Chronic infections are polymicrobial. Gram-negative rods (e.g., *Pseudomonas, Escherichia coli*), anaerobes, and enterococci *may be present in addition to S. aureus* and streptococci.
- Recent hospitalization or use of antibiotics favors growth of fungi and antibiotic-resistant organisms such as methicillin-resistant *S. aureus* and vancomycin-resistant enterococci.

CLINICAL FEATURES AND DIAGNOSIS

Cellulitis

History

Patients may or may not report a history of trauma to the region. Exposure history may provide clues to specific infections, as detailed in Table 11-1. Risk factors such as a history of tinea pedis, diabetes mellitus, surgery for breast cancer with lymph node dissection, saphenous venectomy, or peripheral vascular disease should be determined.

Patients in close contact with other persons who have soft-tissue infections may be at higher risk for methicillin-resistant *S. aureus* (MRSA) infections.

Physical Examination

Fevers and chills occur in a minority of patients but are reported more frequently with *S. pyogenes* infections. The affected area demonstrates erythema without sharply demarcated borders, tenderness, edema, and warmth. Lymphangitis, lymphadenopathy, and abscesses may also be present as well. Cellulitis in patients who have undergone breast cancer surgery with lymph node dissection or saphenous venectomy usually present with evidence of systemic toxicity.

Any potential sites of entry should be noted, and the borders of the affected area should be marked to assess treatment response. Crepitus suggests necrotizing fasciitis and warrants immediate surgical consultation.

Cultures

Cultures are negative in the majority of cases. Only 26% of blood cultures, skin biopsies, and aspiration of the edge of the affected area identify a potential causative organism. One study showed that only 2% of blood cultures are positive in patients with cellulitis. Skin biopsy cultures and cultures of the interdigital spaces in patients with tinea pedis have relatively higher yields.

- Cultures should not be routinely performed.
- Cultures should be reserved for patients with:
    - Fevers, chills, or other systemic manifestations
    - Lack of response to empiric therapy
    - Lymphatic, vascular, or immune compromise
    - Higher risk of MRSA infection
    - Exposures listed in Table 11-1

Diabetic Foot Infection

Assessment of diabetic foot infections should focus on the patient's current condition, predisposing factors for the development of foot ulcers or trauma, presence of vascular insufficiency or neuropathy, wound extent, and microbiology.

Patient

The presence of any systemic signs and symptoms of infection should be noted, including fevers; chills; sweats; evidence of volume depletion such as orthostasis, hypotension, or tachycardia; and changes in mental status. In addition, presence or absence of social support and ability of the patient to care for himself or herself should be determined, because these factors may impact discharge planning.

Laboratory evaluation should include a complete blood count with differential, serum chemistries, creatinine, and blood glucose monitoring.

Predisposing Conditions

Any foot or lower-extremity abnormalities that may result in excessive pressure at the site of the infection should be assessed using physical examination and radiographic imaging.

Arterial or venous insufficiency may predispose to ischemia and gangrene, edema, deep venous thrombosis, poor wound healing, and decreased neutrophil delivery to the wound. Examination of peripheral pulses, ankle to brachial blood pressure index (ABI), and perhaps further evaluation with angiography may be indicated.

The ABI is calculated as follows:

1. Obtain the brachial systolic blood pressure for both upper extremities. Record the higher of the two measurements. This is the brachial pressure.
2. Obtain the systolic blood pressure of the posterior tibial pulse of the affected lower extremity. This is ankle pressure.
3. The ABI is the ankle pressure divided by the brachial pressure.

Physical examination using pinprick, light touch, or vibration may reveal peripheral neuropathy.

Wound Site

The size and depth of the wound, presence of gangrene, and any visible bone, muscle, ligament, or tendon should be noted. Factors that strongly suggest infection include warmth, pain, purulent drainage, induration, and presence of cellulitis, fasciitis, abscess, or osteomyelitis.

The wound site should be cleaned, débrided, and probed for the presence of bone. The practitioner should obtain a culture of the area (see following text) and radiographic imaging such as plain films or MRI.

Infection Severity

The Infectious Diseases Society of America has a system for classifying severity of diabetic foot infections:

- Mild infections possess more than two characteristics of infection (purulence, erythema, pain, tenderness, warmth, or induration), but with an erythematous/cellulitic area less than 2 cm around the wound and limited to the skin and subcutaneous tissue only. No systemic signs or symptoms are present, and no local complications exist.

- Moderate infections have any of the following findings: cellulitis extending more than 2 cm around the wound, lymphangitis, deep tissue abscess, gangrene, spread deeper than the superficial tissues, or involvement of muscle, tendon, joint or bone. No systemic signs or symptoms are present.
- Severe infection is present if a patient has any systemic signs, symptoms, or laboratory abnormalities of metabolic derangement. This may include fevers, chills, hypotension, tachycardia, changes in mental status, electrolyte or acid–base abnormalities, or acute renal insufficiency.

Cultures

Non-infected wounds should not be cultured. Also, patients with mild infection who have not received antibiotics or have not been recently hospitalized may not need cultures. All other patients with diabetic foot infections should have cultures taken of the infected wound. In patients with severe infection, blood cultures should also be performed.

Obtain a wound culture as follows:

- The wound should be cleaned and débrided
- Culture open wounds from the débrided ulcer base using biopsy or curettage with a scalpel blade
- Purulent collections may be cultured using needle aspiration
- Swabs of pus or other fluid exuding from the wound should not be cultured

TREATMENT (Fig. 11-1)

Cellulitis

Hospitalization

Patients with systemic signs and symptoms, such as high fevers or evidence of sepsis, should be admitted for treatment. Patients who do not have systemic manifestations but have severe infection or rapid progression should be considered for inpatient therapy (or outpatient parenteral antibiotics at the very least).

Empiric Antibiotics

Initial choice of empiric antibiotics should cover streptococci and *S. aureus*. Coverage for MRSA should be initiated for patients with severe infection, systemic toxicity, or recent hospitalization or antibiotic exposure. Box 11-1 lists the dosages of commonly used antibiotics.

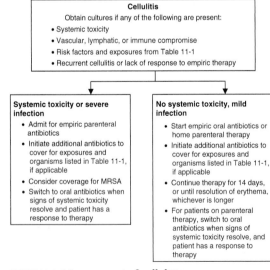

FIGURE 11-1. Management of cellulitis.

Box 11-1. Dosages of Commonly Used Antibiotics

Beta-lactams

- Nafcillin 2 g IV q 4 hr
- Penicillin G 2,000,000 U IV q 4 hr
- Dicloxacillin 500 mg orally q 6 hr
- Amoxicillin-clavulanate 875 mg orally q 12 hr
- Ampicillin-sulbactam 1.53 g IV q 6 hr
- Piperacillin 3 to 4 g IV q 4–6 hr
- Piperacillin-tazobactam 2 g/0.25 g to 4 g/0.5 g IV q 6–8 hr

Carbapenems

- Imipenem-cilastatin 500 mg–1 g IV q 6–8 hr (not to exceed the lower of 50 mg/kg or 4 g/ day)
- Meropenem 1 g IV q 8 hr

Cephalosporins

- Cefazolin 1–2 g IV q 8 hr
- Cefoxitin 1–2 g IV q 6–8 hr
- Cephalexin 500 mg orally q 6 hr
- Cefuroxime 500 mg orally q 12 hr
- Cefuroxime 1.5 g IV q 8 hr (facial *H. influenzae*)
- Ceftazidime 500 mg–1 g IV q 8 hr
- Ceftriaxone 1 g IV q 24 hr

Miscellaneous

- Clindamycin 600 mg IV q 8 hr
- Clindamycin 300 mg orally q 6 hr
- Metronidazole 500 mg orally or IV q 8 hr
- Vancomycin 1 g IV q 12 hr
- Linezolid 600 mg orally q 12 hr

Fluoroquinolones

- Levofloxacin 500 mg orally or IV q 24 hr
- Ciprofloxacin 400 mg IV q 12 hr
- Ciprofloxacin 500 mg orally q 12 hr

Continued

Box 11-1. Dosages of Commonly Used Antibiotics— cont'd

Tetracyclines

- Doxycycline 100 mg orally q 12 hr
- Tetracycline 500 mg orally q 6 hr

Note: Dosages are for patients with normal renal function. Dose adjustments are required for patients with renal insufficiency.

For parenteral therapy, nafcillin or cefazolin may be used. In patients who are allergic to penicillins, other choices include clindamycin or vancomycin. Patients with milder disease may be candidates for oral antibiotics. Dicloxacillin or cephalexin may be used; for patients allergic to beta-lactams, clindamycin or a fluoroquinolone may be given. Antibiotics may be tailored according to culture data, when available.

Parenteral antibiotics should be continued until signs and symptoms of systemic toxicity have resolved, and response to therapy is noted. At this point, changing to an oral antibiotic is reasonable. Total duration of therapy should be 14 days, or until erythema has completely resolved, whichever is longer.

Breast Cancer

Patients who have undergone lymph node dissection as part of breast cancer surgery are usually infected with beta-hemolytic streptococci and, less commonly, *S. aureus*. Empiric therapy remains the same for these patients. However, the cellulitic area should also be monitored for abscess formation, because this would require drainage for successful therapy.

To decrease the risk of recurrence, needlesticks and other potential sources of trauma (e.g., jewelry, blood pressure cuffs) should be minimized on the affected side. Administration of prophylactic antibiotics prior to mammograms is controversial but should be considered.

Water Exposure

Cellulitis developing in the setting of trauma sustained in fresh water may be due to *Aeromonas*, which is resistant to ampicillin. A fluoroquinolone may be initiated in addition to standard empiric therapy.

Cellulitis developing in the setting of salt water trauma warrants coverage for *Vibrio vulnificus*. Coverage with doxycycline should be added to standard empiric therapy.

Hot tub users may have cellulitis due to *Pseudomonas*, and pseudomonal coverage (e.g., ceftazidime) should be added to standard empiric therapy.

Bites

Cat and dog bites may result in *Pasteurella multocida* infection. Human bites may contain many different flora. Amoxicillin-clavulanate or ampicillin-sulbactam should be used as empiric therapy. *P. multocida* is resistant to nafcillin and dicloxacillin.

Facial cellulitis

Facial cellulitis complicating sinusitis or acute otitis media may be due to *H. influenzae*, and a second- or third-generation cephalosporin, such as cefuroxime or ceftriaxone, should be used.

Diabetic Foot Infections

Hospitalization

Patients with severe or limb-threatening infection should be admitted. In addition, patients who lack social support or demonstrate self-neglect should receive inpatient therapy. Some patients with milder infections may require admission for diagnostic testing or observation. Patients with mild infection and no risk factors for antibiotic-resistant organisms or limb ischemia may receive outpatient therapy.

Empiric Antibiotic Choices

For acute mild or moderate non–limb-threatening infections in patients without recent antibiotic exposure or hospitalization, coverage of gram-positive cocci is sufficient. Cephalexin, clindamycin, amoxicillin-clavulanate, or a fluoroquinolone (such as levofloxacin) may be administered orally.

Patients who have been hospitalized recently or have received antibiotics recently for cellulitis, or who are not responding to treatment for gram-positive cocci, should be covered for gram-negative organisms and antibiotic resistant bacteria, such as MRSA. A fluoroquinolone or amoxicillin-clavulanate should be added for gram-negative activity, and vancomycin or linezolid should be initiated to cover MRSA.

More serious chronic infections are likely polymicrobial. Appropriate antibiotic choices must cover gram-positive cocci, gram-negative organisms, and anaerobes. For oral therapy, amoxicillin-clavulanate alone, or a fluoroquinolone plus clindamycin may be used. Parenteral therapy with piperacillin-tazobactam, ticarcillin-clavulanate, or ampicillin-sulbactam monotherapy, or a fluoroquinolone plus clindamycin or metronidazole (to cover anaerobic bacteria) may also be used. Patients with risk factors for resistant organisms should also be covered with vancomycin or linezolid for MRSA.

Patients with severe or limb- or life-threatening infections should be given parenteral therapy with one of the following regimens:

- Piperacillin-tazobactam
- Imipenem-cilastatin
- Clindamycin plus either levofloxacin or ciprofloxacin
- Vancomycin, metronidazole, and ceftazidime.

Treatment should be continued for 2 to 4 weeks. Patients on parenteral therapy may be switched to oral therapy after 1 week if there is clinical improvement.

Antibiotic therapy should be narrowed according to the culture and sensitivity data if the patient is improving.

Surgery

Surgical débridement, drainage of abscesses, revascularization procedures, and amputations may be required for diabetic foot infections. In addition, urgent surgical consultation should be obtained for patients with critical limb ischemia (ABI < 0.5), necrotizing fasciitis, gas gangrene, compartment syndrome, and other potentially life- or limb-threatening complications.

Failure to Respond to Therapy

Patients who do not respond appropriately to the empiric antibiotic regimens described above should be assessed for the following:

- Adequacy of antibiotic coverage
  - If cultures were not obtained or were inadequate, obtaining repeat cultures using curettage or biopsy is indicated
  - If cultures show bacteria that are not covered with the current antibiotics, a change in the regimen may be required
  - If organisms are not identified despite repeat cultures, consider broadening coverage to include gram-negative, anaerobic, and resistant organisms
- Adequacy of surgical therapy
  - If antibiotic coverage is appropriate, consider whether surgical therapy has been adequate
  - Further wound débridement, abscess drainage, or amputation may be required
- Adequacy of wound care
  - The affected lower extremity should be elevated
  - Lower extremity edema should be treated

○ Hyperbaric oxygen or granulocyte colony-stimulating factor (G-CSF) therapy may be considered
- Adequacy of perfusion
  ○ Assess whether arterial or venous insufficiency exists or has been adequately treated
  ○ Imaging with angiography or duplex ultrasonography may be necessary
  ○ Vascular surgery should be consulted if perfusion is compromised

Osteomyelitis

Osteomyelitis should be suspected in any patient with a deep ulcer that overlies a bony area and in patients with a non-healing ulcer despite at least 6 weeks of appropriate antibiotic therapy. Bone that is grossly visible or palpable using a metal probe strongly suggests osteomyelitis.

Patients with chronic ulcers, elevated white count and C-reactive protein as well as either visible or "probe-able" bone should be assumed to have osteomyelitis, and bone biopsy should be considered.

Patients without clinical or laboratory findings highly suggestive of osteomyelitis should have an x-ray examination with plain films.

- If the plain films show classic findings of osteomyelitis (such as soft tissue swelling, periosteal changes, and destruction of bone), bone biopsy to isolate the causative organism should be considered, and the patient should be treated for osteomyelitis
- If plain films are negative for findings of osteomyelitis, the patient should receive 2 weeks of empiric antibiotic therapy and then have another x-ray examination
  ○ If the follow-up films are negative, and the patient continues to improve, treat for soft-tissue infection only
  ○ If the follow-up films demonstrate classic findings of osteomyelitis, bone biopsy

should be considered, and the patient should be treated for osteomyelitis

- If the plain films are not confirmatory, an MRI or bone biopsy may be performed for confirmation
  - If the confirmatory tests do not show osteomyelitis, continue treatment for soft tissue infection
  - If the confirmatory tests demonstrate osteomyelitis, a bone biopsy (if not already done) should be considered and treatment for osteomyelitis administered

Treatment for osteomyelitis should proceed with input from an infectious diseases specialist and an orthopedic surgeon.

REFERENCES

Text Book Chapters

Stevens DL. Cellulitis, pyoderma, abscesses and other skin and subcutaneous infections. In: Cohen J, Powderly WG, and Berkley SF, et al. *Infectious Diseases*, 2nd ed. Philadelphia. Mosby; 2004. pp.133–142.
Handa S. Management of foot ulcer. In: Cohen J, Powderly WG, and Berkley SF, et al. *Infectious Diseases*, 2nd ed. Philadelphia. Mosby; 2004. pp.189–191.

Guidelines

Lipsky BA, Berendt AR, Deery HG, et al. IDSA Guidelines: Diagnosis and Treatment of Diabetic Foot Infections. *Clin Infect Dis* 2004;39:885–910.

CHAPTER 12

Clostridium Difficile Infection

KEY POINTS

1. Recent antibiotic use and inpatient hospitalization are major risk factors for *Clostridium difficile* infection.
2. Cytotoxin assay is the gold standard for diagnosis and detects toxins A and B.
3. ELISA tests have a faster turnaround time but lower sensitivity than the cytotoxin assay. Sending three consecutive samples for ELISA testing may increase the sensitivity of the assay.
4. Some ELISA tests only detect toxin A. Testing for Toxin B is indicated if clinical suspicion is high, and *C. difficile* Toxin A is negative.
5. Patients with high white blood cell count and fever, signs and symptoms of systemic toxicity, or peritoneal signs should be evaluated for toxic megacolon.
6. Initial therapy should begin with metronidazole 500 mg orally, three times daily for 10 to 14 days.
7. Lack of response to metronidazole is not due to antibiotic resistance. Vancomycin 125 mg orally, four times daily, should be used in patients who do not respond to metronidazole.
8. Intracolonic vancomycin and intravenous immunoglobulin therapy are of unproven value at this time.
9. Surgical consultation should be obtained in patients with severe or refractory disease, particularly when complicated by toxic megacolon.

DEFINITION AND EPIDEMIOLOGY
Definition

Clostridium difficile is an anaerobic, spore-forming gram-positive bacillus. *C. difficile* causes a diarrheal infection, which accounts for virtually all cases of pseudomembranous colitis, and 20% of antibiotic-associated diarrhea. The fastidious spores may persist for years in the environment. *C. difficile* produces two toxins, Toxin A and Toxin B, which are cytotoxic and cause colonocyte necrosis. Nontoxin producing strains are not pathogenic.

Incidence

C. difficile diarrhea (CDD) is the most common nosocomial enteric infection. An estimated 300,000 to 3 million new cases occur per year, prolonging inpatient stays by an average of 2 weeks, and increasing hospitalization costs by $6000 to $10,000 per case.

Despite the high inpatient incidence rates, CDD remains an uncommon outpatient problem. The incidence rate is approximately 7.7 cases per 100,000 person-years, or about 20,000 new cases per year. However, many experts believe that CDD is underdiagnosed in the outpatient setting.

Risks

Inpatient Hospitalization

Colonization by *C. difficile* is directly related to the duration of hospital stay. Patients hospitalized for less than 1 week have a colonization rate of 1%, whereas those hospitalized for 4 or more weeks have a colonization rate of greater than 50%.

Sources of spread of *C. difficile* include infected or colonized roommates, carriage on personal items of physicians, and fastidious spores found in the patient's room. Therefore, enteric isolation precautions, room disinfection, and handwashing remain essential for preventing CDD outbreaks (Box 12-1).

Box 12-1. General Principles of *Clostridium difficile* Therapy

General Principles

- Volume resuscitation
- Assess for complications with abdominal imaging if patient has symptoms or signs of systemic toxicity
- Avoid anti-motility or opiate medications
- Discontinue the offending antibiotic. If the antibiotic must be continued, consider switching the antibiotic to another class with a lower risk of causing *C. difficile* diarrhea

Asymptomatic Carrier State

- No indication for medical therapy
- Patients may be at lower risk for the development of symptomatic or recurrent *C. difficile* diarrhea

Antibiotic-Associated Diarrhea without Colitis

- Symptoms usually abate with cessation of the offending antibiotic
- Medical therapy is indicated if antibiotics must be continued or symptoms worsen

C. difficile Colitis with or without Pseudomembranes

- Stop the offending antibiotic, or change to another class with lower risk if antibiotics must be continued
- Medical therapy is indicated

Fulminant Colitis with or without Megacolon

- Stop the offending antibiotic, or change to another class with lower risk if antibiotics must be continued
- Medical therapy is indicated
- Monitor for complications:
  - Development of megacolon
  - Colonic perforation
- Obtain surgical consultation

Antibiotic Use

Antibiotic use is another major risk factor for the acquisition of CDD. The overall risk of CDD is 6.7 cases per 100,000 risk-exposures (defined as 42 days). Antibiotics commonly associated with the development of CDD are clindamycin, ampicillin, amoxicillin, and cephalosporins. Tetracycline, metronidazole, intravenous vancomycin, chloramphenicol, and aminoglycosides have a lower risk for the development of CDD. Other antibiotics carry an intermediate risk for causing CDD.

Rarely, CDD may be associated with the use of chemotherapeutic agents, particularly methotrexate and paclitaxel.

Carrier State and Colonization

Three percent of otherwise healthy adults are carriers of *C. difficile*. Two thirds of patients colonized by *C. difficile* remain asymptomatic. These persons may be at a lower risk for the development of symptomatic CDD (described in more detail in the following text).

Other Risk Factors

Other risk factors for CDD reflect underlying host factors. Elderly or malnourished patients and patients with severe concurrent illness are at higher risk for the development of CDD.

In addition, some studies suggest that the use of proton pump inhibitors may increase the risk of CDD in certain patients.

PATHOGENESIS

Step 1—Exposure to Antibiotics

The first step in the development of CDD is exposure to antibiotics. Antibiotics alter colonic flora, allowing for colonization by *C. difficile*. Although different antibiotics have varying risks for the development of CDD, broad-spectrum antibiotics are usually associated with a higher risk for CDD.

CDD usually develops between days 4 and 9 of an antibiotic course, but has been seen up to 8 weeks following the cessation of therapy.

Step 2—Colonization by *C. difficile*

Fecal–oral acquisition of *C. difficile*, usually during inpatient hospitalization, leads to colonization, with rates as high as 50% after 4 weeks.

Step 3—Development of *C. difficile* Diarrheal Illness:

After colonization, approximately two-thirds of patients become asymptomatic carriers and the remaining one third develop symptomatic CDD. Although the precise reason why some patients develop CDD is unknown, the interactions between *C. difficile* and intrinsic host factors have been implicated.

The development of an antibody response has been shown to be protective against the development of CDD and recurrent CDD. Persons with titers of anti-Toxin A IgG titers less than three ELISA units have an odds ratio of

48 for the development of CDD. Similarly, a systemic IgM response on day 3 and IgG response on day 12 were associated with a decreased risk for recurrent CDD.

CLINICAL FEATURES

Colonization with *C. difficile* results in a range of clinical manifestations, from asymptomatic carrier to fulminant colitis with toxic megacolon (Fig. 12-1).

Asymptomatic Carrier

Approximately 3% of healthy adults and two thirds of patients colonized by *C. difficile* will become asymptomatic carriers. These patients are at lower risk for the development of symptomatic CDD. Although vancomycin may eradicate *C. difficile* in carriers, there is no indication for therapy, because these patients rapidly reacquire the organism.

Antibiotic-Associated Diarrhea

CDD accounts for 20% of all cases of antibiotic-associated diarrhea. In this presentation, colitis and pseudomembranes are absent, diarrhea is mild, and the patient has minimal, if any, systemic symptoms. On examination, patients may report lower abdominal tenderness. Patients will usually respond to withdrawal of the offending antibiotic. If discontinuation of the antibiotic is contraindicated, then switching the antibiotic to one that has a lower risk of CDD should be considered, and medical therapy for CDD should be initiated.

C. difficile Infection with Colitis

Patients have general symptoms of fevers, signs of volume depletion, malaise, and anorexia. Specifically, they may report nausea, moderate

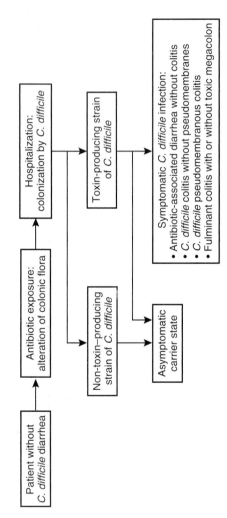

FIGURE 12–1. Colonization by *C. difficile.*

diarrhea with abdominal pain and distension. Physical findings may include abdominal tenderness, and laboratory studies reveal moderate leukocytosis.

Pseudomembranous Colitis

These patients have similar features as those with colitis alone, including systemic signs and symptoms, fevers, volume depletion, and malaise. Physical examination and laboratory tests reveal abdominal tenderness, leukocytosis, and, endoscopically, pseudomembranes (yellowish plaques from 2–10 mm) are noted.

Fulminant Colitis with or without Toxic Megacolon

Fulminant colitis occurs in up to 3% of patients with CDD. Patients present with fevers, profuse diarrhea, severe abdominal pain and cramping, and signs and symptoms of volume depletion. On physical examination, peritoneal signs, such as rebound tenderness, are often present. Laboratory testing reveals marked leukocytosis. A low albumin level may be found if a protein-losing enteropathy is present. Abdominal plain films may reveal complications, including ileus, toxic megacolon, or even frank perforation. Endoscopy is contraindicated in patients with toxic megacolon due to the risk of perforation.

Other Presentations

C. difficile enteritis may occur in patients who have had prior gastrointestinal surgery, particularly partial or total colectomy.

Recurrent CDD may occur in approximately 20% of patients after initial therapy. Relapse of CDD usually occurs after 3 to 12 days following cessation of therapy (mean of 6 days). Patients who have a history of recurrent CDD have a 65% relapse rate. Risk factors for recurrent CDD include number of previous episodes of CDD, lack of immunoglobulin response to Toxin A, continued or additional antibiotic exposure, and renal insufficiency.

CDD may also complicate the course of inflammatory bowel disease (IBD), because patients with IBD have increased exposure to antibiotics as well as sulfasalazine, which may also alter intestinal flora.

DIAGNOSIS

The gold standard for diagnosis is the cytotoxin assay, with a turnaround time of 24 to 48 hours, a sensitivity of 94% to 100%, and specificity of 97%. This assay detects both Toxin A and Toxin B. Limitations to its use include higher cost and longer time to obtain a result.

ELISA testing has a faster turnaround time of 2 to 6 hours and is the preferred method at most institutions. The ELISA test has a sensitivity of 70% to 90% and a specificity close to 99%. The sensitivity may be increased by sending two or three stool samples for testing. A caveat of the ELISA assay is that a laboratory may only test for Toxin A. The number of CDD cases that are positive only for Toxin B range from 1% to 2% in adults to 48% in children. An ELISA assay for Toxin B should be obtained if CDD is strongly suspected and the ELISA assay for Toxin A is negative.

Radiographic imaging is not specific for the diagnosis of CDD, but may provide useful information regarding the extent of disease and the presence of complications. Plain films of the abdomen may reveal ileus, toxic megacolon, or perforation. Abdominal CT imaging may delineate the extent of colonic involvement and provide insight into the complications mentioned previously.

Endoscopic examination in cases of suspected CDD should be reserved for those cases in which:

1. Alternative diagnoses need to be excluded, such as IBD or ischemia

2. Diagnosis must be determined in an urgent or emergent fashion
3. Patient has an ileus, with little stool output available for testing

Due to the risk of perforation, endoscopy should not be performed in patients with toxic megacolon.

TREATMENT

See Box 12-1, Box 12-2, and Table 12-1.

Table 12-1. Treatment for Recurrent *C. difficile* Infection

First Relapse:
Confirm diagnosis of *C. difficile*.
Re-treat with metronidazole 500 mg orally, three times daily for 10–14 days, or vancomycin 125 mg orally, four times daily for 10–14 days

Second Relapse:
Confirm diagnosis of *C. difficile*
Vancomycin tapering and pulsed dose:

Week 1	Vancomycin 125 mg orally, four times daily
Week 2	Vancomycin 125 mg orally, twice daily
Week 3	Vancomycin 125 mg orally, once daily
Week 4	Vancomycin 125 mg orally, every other day
Weeks 5–6	Vancomycin 125 mg orally, every third day

Subsequent Relapses:
One of the following options
1. Vancomycin, 500 mg orally, four times only for 10 days with *Saccharomyces boulardii* 500 mg orally, twice daily for 28 days starting on day 7 of vancomycin treatment
2. Vancomycin 125 mg orally, four times only with Rifampin 600 mg orally, twice daily for 7 days
3. Vancomycin tapering and pulsed dose as described previously, with Cholestyramine 4 g orally, twice daily (can be increased to four times daily)
4. Intravenous immune globulin 300–500 mg/kg every 3 weeks

General Principles

After the diagnosis of CDD is confirmed, the
first step is to provide supportive care. Volume
repletion should be initiated and potential
complications should be addressed. Anti-motility
agents, such as opiates, loperamide, or
diphenoxylate/atropine should not be used
(see Box 12-1).

Toxic megacolon should be suspected in
patients with moderate or severe infection,
decreased bowel sounds, decreasing diarrhea, or
peritoneal signs. In these settings, evaluation with
abdominal plain films or CT scan is indicated. If
megacolon is confirmed, surgical consultation
should be obtained. Patients with moderate or
severe infection without toxic megacolon should
be followed with daily abdominal films for early
detection of megacolon.

Patients with CDD should be placed in a
single room, and enteric pathogen precautions
should be initiated (Box 12-2).

**Box 12-2. American College of Gastroenterology
Guidelines for the Prevention of *Clostridium difficile*
Infection**

1. Limit the use of antimicrobial drugs
2. Wash hands between contact with all patients
3. Use enteric (stool) isolation precautions for
   patients with *C. difficile* diarrhea
4. Wear gloves when in contact with patients
   who have *C. difficile* diarrhea or colitis or with
   their environment
5. Disinfect objects contaminated with *C. difficile*
   with sodium hypochlorite, alkaline glutaralde-
   hyde, or ethylene oxide
6. Educate medical, nursing, and other appropriate staff members about the disease and its
   epidemiology

Cessation of the Precipitating Antibiotic

The first step in the treatment of CDD is cessation of the offending antibiotic. If this is not possible, use of an alternative antibiotic with a lower risk for CDD should be considered. This may be the only intervention necessary in patients with antibiotic-associated diarrhea without colitis. If the antibiotic cannot be stopped, medical therapy should be initiated and treatment should continue for at least 7 to 10 days after the cessation of the culprit antibiotic.

Medical Therapy

First-line therapy for CDD is metronidazole 500 mg orally, three times daily or vancomycin 125 mg orally, four times daily, for a duration of 10 to 14 days. Metronidazole should be used initially in patients with mild to moderate disease because:

- Metronidazole is as effective as vancomycin for the treatment of CDD:
  - A study found that metronidazole 250 mg orally, four times daily was as effective as vancomycin 500 mg orally, four times daily
  - There is no clinically significant resistance to either metronidazole or vancomycin
- Metronidazole is cheaper than vancomycin
- Use of vancomycin may increase selection for vancomycin-resistant enterococci

However, vancomycin should be used as first-line therapy in pregnant or potentially pregnant patients and those intolerant of metronidazole.

Severe or Refractory CDD

Patients who do not respond to metronidazole should be assessed for compliance, presence of alternate diagnoses, exacerbating factors (such as IBD or irritable bowel syndrome) or other potential etiologies. Once these alternative diagnoses have been ruled out, a step-up approach to therapy should be used:

- Vancomycin 125 mg orally, four times daily should be substituted for metronidazole.
- If symptoms do not improve, the vancomycin dose should be doubled every 24–48 hours to a maximum dose of 500 mg orally, four times daily
- Alternatively, metronidazole 500 mg IV three times daily can be given concomitantly with vancomycin 125–500 mg orally, four times daily

For patients with severe CDD who do not respond to this strategy, a case series has suggested possible benefit with intracolonic vancomycin administration:

- 0.5–1 g of vancomycin is placed in 1–2 L of normal saline and given via retention enema every 4–12 hr. This may be continued until clinical improvement is noted.
- For the retention enema, an 18 French Foley catheter with a 30 mL balloon is placed. Following administration of vancomycin, the Foley is clamped for 60 min.

Another case series suggests that a one-time dose of 200 to 300 mg/kg of intravenous immune globulin (IVIG) may be effective for patients with severe, refractory CDD. However, the intracolonic vancomycin and IVIG therapies are derived from uncontrolled, non-randomized case series. Therefore, caution should be exercised in their use until efficacy is confirmed with randomized trials.

Overall, 1% to 3% of patients with CDD require colectomy for refractory disease, toxic megacolon, or colonic perforation. See Box 12-3 for a summary of medical therapy for CDD.

Recurrent CDD

Recurrent CDD occurs in approximately 20% of cases; patients who experience a relapse have up to 65% chance of having additional episodes of CDD. Relapse of CDD is not due to antibiotic resistance.

Box 12-3. Medical Therapy of *Clostridium difficile* Infection

Initial therapy

- Metronidazole 500 mg orally, three times daily for 10–14 days
- Vancomycin 125 mg orally, four times daily for 10–14 days should be used in:
  - Pregnant women
  - Patients intolerant of metronidazole therapy

Severe or Refractory *C. difficile* Infection

- May initiate therapy with metronidazole 500 mg orally, three times daily
- Switch to vancomycin 125 mg orally, four times daily if patient does not respond to metronidazole
  - Increase vancomycin every 48 hr to a maximum dose of 500 mg orally, four times daily
  - May also add metronidazole 500 mg IV every 8 hr if the patient still does not respond
- Unproven therapies:
  - Intracolonic vancomycin, 0.5–1 gm in 1–2 L of normal saline, delivered via an 18 French Foley catheter every 4–12 hr
  - Intravenous immune globulin, a single 200–300 mg/kg/dose
- Surgical therapy—colectomy

First Relapse

1. Confirm the diagnosis of CDD
2. Treat CDD using metronidazole 500 mg orally, three times daily or vancomycin 125 mg orally, four times daily for 10–14 days

Second Relapse

1. Confirm the diagnosis of CDD
2. Begin taper and pulse vancomycin therapy:
   - Week 1: Vancomycin 125 mg orally, four times daily

- Week 2: Vancomycin 125 mg orally, twice dialy
- Week 3: Vancomycin 125 mg orally, once daily
- Week 4: Vancomycin 125 mg orally, every other day
- Weeks 5 and 6: Vancomycin 125 mg orally, every third day

Therapeutic Strategies for Additional Relapses
(Table 12-1)

Saccharomyces boulardii

- Vancomycin, 500 mg orally, four times daily for 10 days
- S. boulardii 500 mg orally, twice daily for 28 days, starting on day 7 of vancomycin treatment
- A randomized, controlled study demonstrated a reduction in the rate of recurrent CDD from 50% to 17% in the S. boulardii group.

Rifampin

Vancomycin 125 mg orally, four times daily for 7 days, with rifampin 600 mg orally, twice daily for 7 days

Cholestyramine

- Vancomycin tapering and pulsed dose as described previously, with
- Cholestyramine 4 gm orally, twice daily (can be increased to four times daily)
- Cholestyramine should be staggered with vancomycin and other medications by 2–3 hr.

Intravenous Immune Globulin (IVIG)

- IVIG given in single doses of 300–500 mg/kg (most commonly, 400 mg/kg), repeated at 3-week intervals.
- Evidence is based on case series data only. Prospective, randomized, controlled studies are lacking. Therefore, there are insuffi-

cient data to recommend IVIG for the treatment of recurrent CDD.

REFERENCES

Textbook Chapters

Bartlett JG. Pseudomembranous enterocolitis and antibiotic-associated diarrhea. In: Feldman M, Friedman LS, and Sleisenger MH, editors. *Sleisenger and Fordtran's Gastrointestinal and Liver Disease*, 7th ed. Philadelphia. WB Saunders; 2002. pp. 1914–1932.

Review Articles

1. Fekety R. Guidelines for the diagnosis and management of *C. difficile*-associated diarrhea and colitis. *Am J Gastroenterol*. 1997;92:739–750.
2. Mylonakis E, Ryan ET, Calderwood SB. *C. difficile*-associated diarrhea. *Arch Intern Med*. 2001;161:525–533.

Treatment

1. Surawicz CM, McFarland LV, Greenberg RN, et al. The search for a better treatment for recurrent *C. difficile* disease: Use of high-dose vancomycin combined with Saccharomyces boulardii. *Clin Infect Dis*. 2000;31:1012–1017.
2. McFarland LV, Elmer GW, Surawicz CM. Breaking the cycle: Treatment strategies for 163 cases of recurrent *Clostridium difficile* disease. *Am J Gastroenterol*. 2002;97:1769–1775.
3. Salcedo J, Keates C, Pothoulakis C, et al. Intravenous immunoglobulin therapy for severe *Clostridium difficile* colitis. *Gut* 1997;41:366–370.
4. Apisarnthanarak A, Razavi B, Mundy L. Adjunctive intracolonic vancomycin for severe *Clostridium difficile* colitis: Case series and review of the literature. *Clin Infect Dis*. 2002;35:690–696.

CHAPTER 13

Community-Acquired Pneumonia

KEY POINTS

1. Aspiration pneumonia accounts for up to 15% of community-acquired pneumonia (CAP) cases, and refers to a lung infection caused by inhalation of oropharyngeal secretions colonized with pathogenic bacteria. If unwitnessed, the diagnosis is inferred when an at-risk patient (nursing home resident, stroke patient) presents with an infiltrate in a characteristic pulmonary location.

2. Aspiration pneumonitis refers to chemical injury to lung caused by inhalation of sterile gastric contents and occurs in patients with altered consciousness.

3. Patients with CAP may present with fever, cough, sputum production, dyspnea, pleurisy, and extrapulmonary symptoms. Chest x-ray usually differentiates CAP from bronchitis and upper respiratory tract infections.

4. On physical examination, the patient may have fever, tachypnea, respiratory distress, hypoxemia, pulmonary crackles, and bronchial breath sounds.

5. Prognostic scoring rules may be used in conjunction with clinical judgment to determine whether a patient with CAP should be hospitalized.

6. Initial testing for patients with CAP requiring hospitalization should include a complete blood count and differential, chemistry panel with renal function and

glucose, assessment of arterial oxygenation, and PA and lateral chest x-ray.

7. Collecting blood and sputum samples in every patient with CAP is controversial, because there is no clear benefit to establishing the causative agent in CAP.

8. The most common CAP pathogens are *Streptococcus pneumoniae, Mycoplasma pneumoniae, Chlamydia pneumoniae*, and *Legionella* species.

9. Presenting features of CAP do not predict the causative agent.

10. Approximately 20% of *S. pneumoniae* are penicillin-resistant and one third are macrolide-resistant. Fluoroquinolone resistance is low in the United States.

11. Infectious Diseases Society of America recommends a beta-lactam plus a macrolide or fluoroquinolone monotherapy as empiric treatment for patients with CAP admitted to the general medical ward.

12. Patients admitted to the intensive care unit should receive coverage for *S. pneumoniae, Legionella*, and possibly *Pseudomonas*.

13. The optimum duration of antibiotic administration is unknown (7–10 days is reasonable in most cases).

14. Even with appropriate antibiotic use, fevers may take up to 72 hours to fully resolve. Persistent fevers or declining clinical status should prompt an evaluation for complications or worsening pneumonia.

15. Pulmonary infiltrates can take weeks or months to fully resolve following treatment.

16. Aspiration pneumonitis does not usually require antibiotic therapy unless the patient is at risk for bacterial colonization of the gastric contents or

the symptoms do not resolve within 48 hours of the event.

17. Therapy for aspiration pneumonia includes a swallowing evaluation and antibiotics with activity against gram-negative bacteria. Anaerobic coverage is appropriate in some settings (e.g., a lung abscess or severe periodontal disease).

18. Preventive measures against CAP include smoking cessation and administration of the polysaccharide pneumococcal and inactivated influenza vaccines.

DEFINITIONS

Nosocomial pneumonia: Hospital-acquired pneumonia starting at least 48 to 72 hours after admission.

Aspiration pneumonia: Lung infection caused by inhalation of oropharyngeal secretions that are colonized with pathogenic bacteria.

Aspiration pneumonitis: Chemical injury to lung caused by inhalation of sterile gastric contents.

EPIDEMIOLOGY

An estimated 4 million cases of community-acquired pneumonia (CAP) occur annually in the United States, accounting for at least 600,000 hospital admissions. CAP is the sixth leading cause of death. The mortality rate for hospitalized CAP patients is approximately 1 in 10 but this rate is higher in specific populations (e.g., nursing home residents) and approaches 40% in the severely ill who require admission to the intensive care unit.

Aspiration Pneumonia

Aspiration pneumonia accounts for up to 15% of CAP cases and is common among nursing home residents. The risk of aspiration pneumonia is higher in the elderly and patients with dysphagia, stroke, or critical illness and lower in patients without teeth. Usually, the episode of aspiration is not witnessed; the diagnosis is inferred when patients at risk for aspiration present with an infiltrate in a characteristic pulmonary location (posterior upper lobe or apical lower lobe segments from recumbent aspiration, and basal lower lobe segments from upright or semi-recumbent aspiration). Patients with aspiration pneumonia have clinical features similar to those of patients with CAP but have a higher incidence of pulmonary cavitation and abscess formation.

Early studies identified anaerobic organisms as the predominant pathogens in patients with aspiration pneumonia, but this has not been confirmed in recent studies.

Aspiration Pneumonitis

Aspiration pneumonitis occurs in patients with altered consciousness (e.g., seizures, drug overdose, and anesthesia). The aspirated gastric contents are usually sterile but the acidity burns the lung, causing an intense inflammatory reaction. Bacterial infection may subsequently develop, but the prevalence of this complication is unknown. Infection likely plays some role if the gastric contents are colonized with pathogenic organisms (e.g., gastroparesis, enteral feedings, and ant-acid therapy raise the gastric pH and increase the risk of bacterial colonization).

Aspiration pneumonitis has a broad spectrum of presentation, ranging from cough or wheeze to cyanosis, shortness of breath, hypoxemia, hypotension, acute respiratory distress syndrome, and death.

Causes of Community-Acquired Pneumonia

Most cases of CAP are limited to a few key organisms (Box 13-1), although in most cases the cause of the pneumonia is not identified. *S. pneumoniae* (pneumococcus) accounts for approximately two thirds of all cases of bacteremic pneumonia. Other common pathogens include *M. pneumoniae*, *C. pneumoniae*, and *Legionella* species, which have been reported to cause "atypical" pneumonia (pneumonia that does not present with classic signs and symptoms).

Box 13-1. Some Causative Agents of Community-Acquired Pneumonia

Bacterial

Streptococcus pneumoniae

Haemophilus influenzae

Mycoplasma pneumoniae

Legionella species

Chlamydia pneumoniae

Chlamydia psittaci

Coxiella burnetii

Staphylococcus aureus

Pseudomonas aeruginosa

Enteric gram-negatives

Anaerobes

Viral

Influenza virus

Respiratory syncytial virus

Parainfluenza virus

Adenovirus

Coronavirus

Adapted from File TM. Community-acquired pneumonia. *Lancet.* 2003;362:1991–2001.

In the past, the presenting signs and symptoms of pneumonia were thought to predict the causative agent, but we now know this to be untrue—there is a wide spectrum of presentation for each organism that is known to cause CAP, and these pathogens cannot be distinguished based only on symptoms, clinical signs, and findings on chest x-ray.

SYMPTOMS AND SIGNS

Immunocompetent adults presenting with pneumonia may have fever ($\sim 80\%$), cough ($> 90\%$), sputum production ($\sim 66\%$), dyspnea ($\sim 66\%$), and pleuritic chest pain ($\sim 50\%$). However, these symptoms may also occur in patients with bronchitis or upper respiratory tract infections. Therefore, symptoms at presentation do not reliably distinguish between CAP and other respiratory illnesses. Bronchitis and upper respiratory tract infections are usually caused by viruses and can almost always be differentiated from pneumonia using chest x-ray. One caveat is that the chest x-ray may be normal in patients with CAP who are dehydrated. In this setting, the infiltrate should become visible following adequate hydration.

Extrapulmonary symptoms, including gastrointestinal symptoms, headache, myalgias, and arthralgias, occur in up to one third of CAP patients.

Physical exam findings depend on the severity of the infection. The patient may have fever, tachypnea, hypoxemia, pulmonary crackles, bronchial breath sounds, and respiratory distress with accessory respiratory muscle use.

Laboratory Data

Initial laboratory testing for patients with CAP requiring hospital admission should include:

1. Complete blood count (with differential) and chemistry panel, including assessment of renal function and glucose
2. Blood cultures (controversial; see following text)
3. PA and lateral chest x-ray, which may show a lobar (occurring in one lobe of the lung) or segmental pulmonary infiltrate, patchy or diffuse lung infiltrates, or pleural effusion. The "air bronchogram sign" occurs when dense lung consolidation delineates air in the intrapulmonary bronchi, which are not normally visualized on chest x-ray. This sign confirms the presence of lung consolidation. The chest x-ray is also useful for ruling out complications, such as pneumothorax, abscesses, and empyema.
4. Sputum for gram stain and culture from a deep cough (controversial; see following text). If appropriate, also test the sputum for tuberculosis, *Legionella*, fungi, and viruses.
5. Assessment of arterial oxygenation (arterial blood gas or pulse oximetry)
6. Thoracentesis to rule out empyema if there is an effusion measuring > 10 mm on lateral decubitus chest x-ray

Other tests that may be appropriate (depending on the clinical circumstances) include:

1. Urine antigen assay for *L. pneumoniae* serogroup 1. This test is appropriate for (a) hospitalized patients with an unusual presentation of pneumonia, (b) patients with an unusual pneumonia admitted to the intensive care unit during a *Legionella* epidemic, and (c) patients who fail to respond to a beta-lactam antibiotic.
2. Urine antigen assay for *S. pneumoniae*. This test can be used as an adjunct to blood and sputum cultures, with the potential advantage of a rapid turnaround time.

There is no well-documented benefit for establishing the causative agent in CAP. Therefore, collection of blood and sputum samples in all CAP patients is controversial. Sputum samples are also limited by the ability of the patient to produce a good specimen and the experience of the person interpreting the Gram stain. Nonetheless, these samples may be useful for directing therapy if the patient fails to respond to empiric treatment. Ideally, sputum and blood samples should be collected prior to antibiotic administration, but antibiotic therapy should never be delayed because early treatment is important for the outcome of CAP.

TREATMENT

Should the Patient with CAP be Admitted to the Hospital?

If you are on the inpatient medicine service, this decision has already been made. However, you may be involved in the decision-making process during a rotation through the emergency department or if you see a patient with CAP in clinic. Recognized risk factors for increased mortality in CAP include advanced age and co-morbidities, such as cancer and heart failure. The decision to admit relies on clinical judgment, although there are also prognostic scoring rules that can support this decision. The most widely used and rigorously studied prediction rule is the Pneumonia PORT (Pneumonia Outcomes Research Team) Severity Index (PSI), which stratifies patients into one of five categories using a point system based on several variables at the time of presentation (Fig. 13-1). An easy-to-use version is available on the internet at *http://ncemi.org*. The higher the score, the higher the 30-day mortality rates, the longer the length of stay, the higher the risk of admission to the intensive care unit, and the higher the risk of readmission to the hospital. The risk for

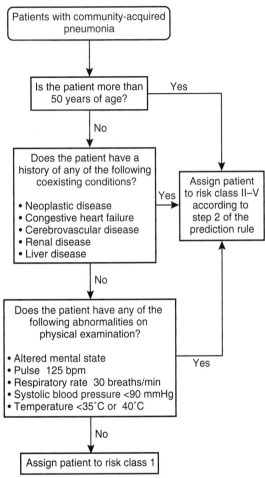

FIGURE 13–1. Calculation of the Pneumonia PORT (Pneumonia Outcomes Research Team) Severity Index (PSI).

Continued

Point Scoring System for Assignment to Risk Classes II, III, IV, and V (sum each applicable characteristic to calculate the total score).

Age	
Men	Age (years)
Women	Age (years) − 10
Nursing home resident	**+ 10**
Co-morbidities	
Neoplastic disease	+ 30
Liver disease	+ 20
Congestive heart failure	+ 10
Cerebrovascular disease	+ 10
Renal disease	+ 10
Physical exam findings	
Altered mental status	+ 20
Respiratory rate $\geq$ 30/min	+ 20
Systolic blood pressure < 90 mm Hg	+ 20
Temperature < 35°C or $\geq$ 40°C	+ 15
Pulse $\geq$ 125/min	+ 10
Laboratory findings	
Arterial pH < 7.35	+ 30
Blood urea nitrogen $\geq$ 11 mmol/L	+ 20
Sodium < 130 mmol/L	+ 20
Glucose $\geq$ 250 mg/dL	+ 10
Hematocrit < 30%	+ 10
pO_2 < 60 mm Hg or O_2 sat < 90%	+ 10
Pleural effusion	+ 10

Neoplastic disease = any cancer (except basal- or squamous-cell skin cancer) active at the time of presentation or diagnosed within 1 year of presentation

Liver disease = clinical or histologic diagnosis of cirrhosis or other chronic liver disease.

FIGURE 13–1. *Continued*

Stratification of Risk Score (based on the previous algorithms)			
Risk Class	Total Score	Recommended Site of Treatment	Mortality Range (%)
I	0	Outpatient	0.1
II	≤ 70	Outpatient	0.6
III	71–90	Outpatient	0.9–2.8
IV	91–130	Inpatient	8.2–9.3
V	> 130	Inpatient	27.0–29.2

From Fine MJ, *et al.* A prediction rule to identify low-risk patients with community-acquired pneumonia. *N Engl J Med.* 1997;336:243–250. Copyright © 1997 Massachusetts Medical Society. All rights reserved. Adapted with permission, 2005.

FIGURE 13–1. *Continued*

death ranges from 0.1% to 2.8% for classes I to III, 8.2% to 9.3% for class IV, and 27% to 31% for class V. Therefore, the Infectious Diseases Society of America recommends home care for risk classes I to III only. Patients with low PORT scores may fail outpatient treatment because of preexisting conditions, such as social or psychiatric problems, inability to take oral medication, or acute hypoxemia. Therefore, an assessment for factors that may compromise successful outpatient therapy for CAP should occur prior to calculation of the PORT score. In other words, prediction rules might oversimplify the interpretation of important variables. Therefore, these scoring systems should not take the place of clinical judgment.

Medications

Drug-Resistant *S. pneumoniae*

Drug-resistant *S. pneumoniae* is on the rise— 20% of *S. pneumoniae* are penicillin-resistant and approximately one third are macrolide-resistant. Fluoroquinolone resistance is low in the United States. Risk factors for penicillin

Box 13-2. Risk Factors for Drug-Resistant *Strepto-coccus pneumoniae*

Penicillin-Resistance*

Age > 65 years

Treatment with a beta-lactam within 3 months

Medical co-morbidities

Alcoholism

Immunosuppression

Exposure to a child in a daycare center

Levofloxacin-Resistance[†]

Nursing home resident

Nosocomial infection

Previous exposure to a fluoroquinolone

Chronic obstructive pulmonary disease

---

*Adapted from File TM. Community-acquired pneumonia. *Lancet.* 2003;362:1991-2001.
[†] Adapted from Ho PL, et al. Risk factors for acquisition of levo-floxacin-resistant *Streptococcus pneumoniae:* a case control study. *Clin Infect Dis.* 2001;32:701–707.

and fluoroquinolone resistance are listed in Box 13-2.

Guidelines for Empiric Treatment

The Infectious Diseases Society of America recommends a beta-lactam plus a macrolide, or fluoroquinolone monotherapy for the empiric treatment of CAP requiring admission to the general medical ward (Table 13-1). These regimens have been shown to reduce mortality when compared to cephalosporin monotherapy. Patients admitted to the intensive care unit with CAP should receive coverage for *S. pneumoniae*, *Legionella*, and possibly *Pseudomonas* (see Table 13-1). Risk factors for *Pseudomonas* infection include structural lung disease (e.g., bronchiectasis) and recent hospitalization

Table 13-1. Recommendations for Empirical Inpatient Treatment of Community-Acquired Pneumonia for Patients Admitted to the Medical Ward and Intensive Care Unit

	Examples with Dosing*
Medical Ward	
Anti-pneumococcal fluoroquinolone	Levofloxacin 500 mg q24h OR gatifloxacin 400 mg q24h OR moxifloxacin 400 mg q24h
β-lactam with macrolide	Ceftriaxone 1–2 g IV q24h OR cefotaxime 1–2 g IV q8h OR ampicillin/sulbactam 1.5–3 g IV q6h PLUS Azithromycin 500 mg IV q24h OR clarithromycin 250 mg PO q12h
Intensive Care Unit	
If pseudomonas is not a concern: β-lactam plus macrolide or fluoroquinolone monotherapy	**No beta-lactam allergy:** Ceftriaxone 1–2 g IV q24h OR cefotaxime 2 g IV q4–8h OR ampicillin/sulbactam 1.5–3 g IV q6h OR piperacillin/tazobactam 3.375 g IV q6h PLUS Azithromycin 500 mg IV q24h **Beta-lactam allergy:** Levofloxacin 500 mg q24h± clindamycin 600 mg IV q8h
If pseudomonas is a concern (see text) Anti-pseudomonal agent and anti-pseudomonal fluoroquinolone	**No beta-lactam allergy:** Pipercillin/tazobactum 3.375 g IV q6h OR cefepime 1–2 g IV q12h AND Ciprofloxacin 400 mg IV q8–12h OR levofloxacin 500 mg q24h **Beta-lactam allergy:** Aztreonam 1–2 g IV q6–12h AND levofloxacin 500 mg q24h

Adapted with Permission from Mandell LA, Bartlett JG, Dowell SF, et al. Update of practice guidelines for the management of community-acquired pneumonia in immunocompetent adults. *Clin Infect Dis.* 2003;37:1405–1433. Copyright © 2003 The University of Chicago Press and the Infectious Diseases Society of America.
*Dosages assume normal renal function. Fluoroquinolone dosages are IV or oral, unless otherwise indicated.

(especially if the prior hospital stay included time in the intensive care unit).

Additional Recommendations Regarding Antibiotic Use

If a causative organism is identified based on sputum or blood sample results, the empiric antibiotic regimen should be switched to a narrow spectrum agent based on susceptibilities. This practice should reduce selective pressures for bacterial resistance.

The optimum duration of antibiotic administration is unknown, but most physicians treat for 7 to 10 days based on patient co-morbidities and response to treatment. With appropriate antibiotic use, fevers will trend downwards but may take up to 72 hours to fully resolve. Persistent fevers or worsening clinical status should prompt an evaluation for worsening pneumonia (repeat chest x-ray and possibly a CT scan) or complications, such as an empyema or metastatic infection (meningitis, septic arthritis, pericarditis, and peritonitis).

Therapy for Aspiration Pneumonitis

After a witnessed aspiration event, the upper airway should be suctioned. Prophylactic antibiotics are frequently used but are generally not indicated (at least initially) in the majority of patients with aspiration pneumonitis because the antibiotics may select for resistant organisms in patients with uncomplicated chemical pneumonitis. Antibiotic therapy is appropriate if the aspiration pneumonitis does not resolve within 48 hours of the aspiration event or if the patient is likely to have bacterial colonization of the gastric contents (e.g., small bowel obstruction or use of antacids or proton pump inhibitors). In this setting, broad-spectrum agents are recommended. Anaerobic coverage is not routinely needed. A reasonable treatment plan is

levofloxacin 500 mg daily or intravenous ceftriaxone 1 to 2 g daily (dosages assume normal
renal function). Glucocorticoids have no proven
benefit.

Therapy for Aspiration Pneumonia

Crude assessment of the cough and gag reflexes
unreliably identifies patients at risk for aspiration. Rather, a comprehensive swallowing evaluation is required (preferably a swallow study
with concurrent speech therapy evaluation).
A soft diet should be started if swallowing dysfunction is detected and the patient should be
taught strategies to lower the risk of aspiration,
such as reducing the bite size, swallowing
repeatedly, and keeping the chin tucked while
eating.

Percutaneous endoscopic gastrostomy (PEG)
tubes are no longer routinely used in patients at
high-risk for aspiration, because PEG tubes have
not been shown to alter mortality in this population.

Antibiotics are standard of care for patients
with aspiration pneumonia. Therapy should
generally include activity against gram-negative
organisms. Levofloxacin 500 mg daily is a reasonable treatment option (dosage assumes normal renal function). Anaerobic coverage (e.g., IV
clindamycin 600 mg three times daily or metronidazole 500 mg three times daily) should be
added if there is a lung abscess, necrotizing
pneumonia, severe periodontal disease, or putrid
sputum.

WHEN IS THE CAP PATIENT READY FOR DISCHARGE?

The Infectious Diseases Society of America
recommends that the patient have no more than
one of the following characteristics during the
24 hours preceding hospital discharge (unless
this represents the patient's baseline status):

1. Temperature $> 37.8°$ C ($> 100°$ F)
2. Pulse > 100 bpm
3. Respiratory rate > 24 breaths / min
4. Systolic blood pressure < 90 mm Hg
5. Blood oxygen saturation $< 90\%$
6. Inability to maintain oral intake

Pulmonary infiltrates may take up to several weeks or even months to fully resolve after successful treatment of CAP (especially in smokers, the elderly, and patients with underlying lung disease).

PREVENTION

The following prevention measures should be addressed with every CAP patient:

1. Encourage smoking cessation, if applicable.
2. Administer the polysaccharide pneumococcal vaccine to:
   (a) Patients 65 years and older (redose if the person was vaccinated before the age of 65 years and 5 or more years have elapsed since the initial vaccination).
   (b) Patients younger than 65 years who live in a chronic care facility or who have a compromised immune system, diabetes mellitus, alcoholism, chronic pulmonary, liver, or cardiovascular disease (redose when the patient is over the age of 65 years and 5 or more years have elapsed since the initial vaccination).
3. Administer the inactivated influenza vaccine to:
   (a) Patients 50 years of age and older
   (b) Residents of chronic care facilities or patients with diabetes mellitus, immuno-suppression, or chronic pulmonary, renal, or cardiovascular disease

The inactivated influenza vaccine can be given to patients with a minor respiratory illness but administration should be delayed in patients with acute febrile illness until symptoms have mostly resolved. Patients with a history of ana-phylaxis to hens' eggs should not be given the vaccine nor should those who developed Guillain-Barré syndrome from a prior influenza vaccine.

REFERENCES

Review articles

1. File TM. Community-acquired pneumonia. *Lancet* 2003;362:1991–2001.
2. Prevention and control of influenza. Recommendations of the Advisory Committee on Immunization Practices (ACIP). *MMWR Morb Mortal Wkly Rep.* 2004;53(RR-6):1–40.
3. Marik PE. Aspiration pneumonitis and aspiration pneumonia. *N Engl J Med.* 2001;344:665–671.
4. Halm EA, Teirstein AS. Management of community-acquired pneumonia. *N Engl J Med.* 2002;347:2039–2045.
5. Stout JE, Yu VL. Legionellosis. *N Engl J Med.* 1997;337:682–687.

Signs, Symptoms, and Prognosis

1. Fine MJ, Auble TE, Yealy DM, et al. A prediction rule to identify low-risk patients with community-acquired pneumonia. *N Engl J Med.* 1997;336:243–250.
2. Metlay JP, Fine MJ. Testing strategies in the initial management of patients with community-acquired pneumonia. *Ann Intern Med.* 2003;138:109–118.

Treatment

1. Mandell LA, Bartlett JG, Dowell SF, et al. Update of practice guidelines for the management of community-acquired pneumonia in immunocompetent adults. *Clin Infect Dis.* 2003;37:1405–1433.

2. Niederman MS, Mandell LA, Anzueto A, et al. Guidelines for the management of adults with community-acquired pneumonia. Diagnosis, assessment of severity, antimicrobial therapy, and prevention. *Am J Respir Crit Care Med*. 2001;163:1730–1754.

3. Mandell LA, Marrie TJ, Grossman RF, et al, Canadian Community-Acquired Pneumonia Working Group. Canadian guidelines for the initial management of community-acquired pneumonia: An evidence-based update by the Canadian Infectious Diseases Society and the Canadian Thoracic Society. *Clin Infect Dis*. 2000;31:383–421.

Urinary Tract Infections

KEY POINTS

1. Urinary tract infections occur more commonly in women than in men, mainly due to anatomic differences.

2. Patients with acute cystitis may complain of dysuria, increased urinary frequency or urgency. Fever, nausea, vomiting, and flank pain (costovertebral tenderness) are signs and symptoms of an upper urinary tract infection, such as pyelonephritis, renal abscess, or perinephric abscess.

3. Urinalysis and urine dipstick are sufficient for patients with uncomplicated acute cystitis (young women without comorbidities). Urine culture should be reserved for patients with complicated urinary tract infections, patients not responding to empiric therapy, or patients with upper urinary tract infections.

4. Empiric therapy of uncomplicated acute cystitis should begin with trimethoprim-sulfamethoxazole 160 mg/800 mg twice daily for 3 days.

5. Empiric therapy of acute pyelonephritis or complicated urinary tract infections should begin with a fluoroquinolone, such as ciprofloxacin 500 mg orally twice daily or levofloxacin 500 mg orally daily.

6. A renal or perinephric abscess should be suspected in patients who do not improve, or who deteriorate despite adequate medical therapy.

DEFINITION

Cystitis (bladder infection or inflammation) may occur with or without pyelonephritis (infection of the kidney[s]). Acute cystitis in a young woman without comorbidities is an uncomplicated urinary tract infection (UTI). The episode is considered a complicated UTI when the risk of treatment failure is higher (e.g., patients with pyelonephritis, diabetes mellitus, immunosuppression, urinary tract abnormality, male sex, older age, urinary tract instrumentation, or hospital-acquired infection).

EPIDEMIOLOGY

UTIs account for 8 million physician visits and over 100,000 hospitalizations per year. Women are affected by 0.5 UTIs per year in their 20s and roughly 0.1 infections per year in their 30s. Up to 60% of women report being affected by a UTI at some time in their lives. Among postmenopausal women, studies report an incidence of 0.07 cases per person-year. The incidence of UTIs in men is significantly lower (5–8 cases per 10,000 persons).

Escherichia coli is the most common cause of UTIs, accounting for 80% to 90% of cases. *Staphylococcus saprophyticus* is the next most common pathogen, accounting for 10% to 20% of cases. A small minority of cases are caused by *Proteus*, *Klebsiella*, or enterococci. Complicated UTIs are usually caused by *Pseudomonas aeruginosa*, resistant gram-negative organisms, and fungi. More than 90% of cases of uncomplicated cystitis are monomicrobial, whereas up to 30% of cases of complicated urinary tract infections may be polymicrobial.

UTIs are the most common nosocomial infection, with an incidence of 2 cases per 100 patients discharged from the hospital.

Most cases of hospital-acquired UTIs are associated with urinary catheterization.

Renal cortical abscesses (renal carbuncle) are usually due to hematogenous seeding of bacteria. *S. aureus* is the causative organism in 90% of cases. Renal cortical abscesses tend to be unilateral and occur in the right kidney 63% of the time. Men are affected three times more often than women.

Renal corticomedullary abscesses, in contrast, are usually caused by an ascending UTI with gram-negative bacteria such as *E. coli*, *Proteus*, and *Klebsiella*. Men and women are affected equally. Severe infections may penetrate the renal capsule and cause a perinephric abscess. Patients with urinary tract abnormalities are at higher risk for the development of renal corticomedullary abscesses.

Perinephric abscesses develop from rupture of a renal abscess; therefore, both conditions share many of the same risk factors. Roughly 25% of perinephric abscesses occur in patients with diabetes.

PATHOGENESIS

Colonization of the vaginal introitus by pathogenic fecal flora, followed by introduction of the pathogens into the urinary system cause UTIs. Sexual intercourse and intercourse with spermicide-containing contraceptives, history of multiple UTIs, and presence of diabetes mellitus are the major risk factors for the development of UTIs.

Men experience far fewer cases of UTIs than do women because of the longer urethra, decreased colonization of the peri-urethral region, and secretion of antibacterial substances in prostatic fluid.

In cases of catheter-associated urinary tract infections, bacteria may gain access to the bladder via the catheter lumen or along the outside of the catheter.

CLINICAL FEATURES AND DIAGNOSIS

History

The predominant symptom of cystitis is dysuria (pain when urinating), in association with increased urinary frequency, suprapubic pain, or hematuria. It is important to rule out other causes of dysuria, including urethritis caused by sexually transmitted diseases (STD), such as gonorrhea or chlamydia. Patients with urethral discharge, recent new sexual partner, or sexual partner with urethral symptoms should be investigated for urethritis caused by an STD. Vaginitis may also cause dysuria. Patients with dyspareunia, vaginal discharge, vaginal pruritus, or dysuria without associated increased urinary frequency should be worked up for vaginitis. Women with dysuria, increased urinary frequency, and no vaginal symptoms have a >90% likelihood of having acute cystitis.

Pyelonephritis or other upper UTIs should be suspected in patients with fevers, chills, nausea, vomiting, flank pain, and other systemic signs or symptoms. Fevers greater than 100° F (37.8° C) correlate well with the presence of pyelonephritis instead of cystitis.

Renal and perinephric abscesses may present with fevers, chills, and back, abdominal or flank pain. Patients with renal cortical abscesses may not report urinary symptoms because these abscesses rarely communicate with the urinary system.

Physical Examination

Patients with acute cystitis may have suprapubic tenderness. A pelvic examination (with testing for gonorrhea and chlamydia) should be performed if urethritis or vaginitis is suspected. Patients with upper UTI may have fever, tachycardia, and costovertebral angle tenderness.

Laboratory Tests

Urinalysis and Urine Dipsticks

More than 10 white blood cells per microliter in the urine are highly suggestive of a UTI. White blood cell casts suggest upper UTI. The presence of hematuria supports the diagnosis of UTI; hematuria is not found in urethritis or vaginitis.

Leukocyte esterase testing on urinary dipsticks has a sensitivity of up to 96%, and a specificity of up to 98% for the detection of white blood cells in the urine. The nitrite test detects the presence of Enterobacteriaceae, but may be falsely negative in patients with lower numbers of bacteria (<10,000 cfu/mL). The nitrite test is most accurate if applied to the first urine collected in the morning (prolonged exposure to bacteria is required to convert nitrates to nitrites). The nitrite test should not be used to rule out acute pyelonephritis because the test has lower sensitivity for this condition (35%–80%) and cannot detect non-nitrite-producing bacteria.

Urine Culture

Urine cultures should be reserved for patients likely to have complicated UTIs, patients failing initial anti-microbial therapy, patients with atypical symptoms, and patients with upper UTIs, including acute pyelonephritis. Although the standard cutoff for a positive urine culture is > 100,000 cfu/mL, in women with pyuria and UTI symptoms, a urine culture is positive if the bacterial count exceeds 100 cfu/mL.

Studies have shown that over one half of patients with typical UTI symptoms, pyuria, and negative cultures have *Chlamydia trachomatis* infection. The remainder of women do not have any identifiable organism but may still respond to standard therapy for acute cystitis.

Blood Culture

Up to 20% of patients with pyelonephritis will have a positive blood culture.

Renal and Perinephric Abscesses

Patients with renal cortical abscesses may not have a positive urinalysis or urine culture unless the abscess communicates with the urinary tract. Blood cultures are rarely positive. Renal corticomedullary abscesses may be diagnosed by CT scanning or ultrasound. (CT scanning is the most sensitive diagnostic technique.) Perinephric abscesses may be visualized on CT or MRI scanning. MRI may provide better delineation of adjacent tissue and organ involvement.

Further Evaluation

Men with urinary tract infections should have imaging of the urinary tract with ultrasound, KUB plain film, or intravenous urogram.

TREATMENT (Box 14-1)

Uncomplicated Acute Cystitis

A 3-day course of trimethoprim (TMP), trimethoprim-sulfamethoxazole (TMP-SMX), or a fluoroquinolone (FQ) such as ofloxacin, ciprofloxacin, or norfloxacin should be used as empiric therapy for uncomplicated acute cystitis. These regimens achieve an eradication rate >90%. Due to lower costs, a 3-day course of double-strength TMP-SMX should be the initial drug of choice for empiric therapy of uncomplicated acute cystitis in women. FQ should be used as initial empiric therapy if the patient is allergic to TMP-SMX, has used TMP-SMX within the last 3 months (may increase the chance of TMP-SMX resistance), or lives in an area where >20% of E. coli isolates are resistant to TMP-SMX.

Box 14-1. Common Medication Dosages

Acute Cystitis

- Trimethoprim–sulfamethoxazole 160 mg/800 mg orally twice a day for 3 days
- Trimethoprim 300 mg orally daily for 3 days
- Levofloxacin 250 mg orally daily for 3 days
- Norfloxacin 400 mg orally every 12 hr for 3 days
- Ciprofloxacin 250 mg orally twice a day (or 500 mg orally daily) for 3 days
- Macrobid 100 mg orally twice a day for 7 days

Complicated Acute Cystitis:

- Empiric therapy: Fluoroquinolone at the above listed doses for 1–2 weeks

Antibiotics in Pregnancy:

Do not use:

- Trimethoprim—anti-folate effects, and potential megaloblastic anemia
- Sulfonamides—kernicterus
- Tetracycline—stains teeth of fetus/infant. May be hepatotoxic to mother
- Fluoroquinolones—arthropathy

Acute Pyelonephritis:

- Ciprofloxacin 500 mg orally every 12 hr, or 400 mg IV every 12 hr
- Levofloxacin 500 mg orally daily or 500 mg IV daily
- Gatifloxacin 400 mg orally daily or 400 mg IV daily
- Norfloxacin 400 mg orally every 12 hr
- Gentamicin 5 mg/kg IV daily with ampicillin 1–2 g IV every 6 hr. Use ampicillin for suspected enterococci infection

Other Medications:

- Nafcillin 1–2 g IV every 4–6 hr
- Oxacillin 1–2 g IV every 4–6 hr
- Piperacillin 3–4 g IV every 4–6 hr
- Cefazolin 1–2 g IV every 8 hr
- Cefotaxime 1 g IV every 8 hr
- Ceftriaxone 1 g IV every 24 hr
- Ceftazidime 1–2 g IV every 8 hr
- Vancomycin 1 g IV every 12 hr
- Tobramycin 5 mg/kg/day IV
- Fluconazole 50–100 mg orally daily
- Fluconazole 50–400 mg/day IV

Note: Dosages are for patients with normal renal function. Dose adjustments may be required for patients with renal impairment.

Any of the preceding antibiotics has activity against *E. coli* (although resistance to TMP-SMX is rising). TMP-SMX and FQ have activity against *S. saprophyticus.*

Single-dose therapy is not recommended, because it has inferior eradication rates. For uncomplicated UTI, 7-day therapy has eradication rates equivalent to those of 3-day therapy. Beta-lactams have lower eradication rates than TMP, TMP-SMX, or FQ. Nitrofurantoin as a 3-day course appears to have inferior eradication rates when compared to a 3-day course of TMP-SMX.

Urinary tract analgesia may be achieved with the use of phenazopyridine 200 mg orally three times a day in patients with significant dysuria.

Complicated Acute Cystitis

Patients who are elderly, diabetic, immunocompromised, pregnant, institutionalized, hospitalized, or who have an indwelling urinary catheter, a history of recent antibiotic use, or a urinary system abnormality are at higher risk for treatment failure. Pathogens seen in patients with complicated UTIs include *E. coli*, *Proteus*, *Klebsiella*, enterococci, staphylococci, and fungi. Evaluation of these patients should always include urine culture and antibiotic sensitivity testing.

Because of an increased resistance rate to commonly used antibiotics, the first-line empiric therapy for patients with complicated acute cystitis is a fluoroquinolone antibiotic, such as levofloxacin or ciprofloxacin. Moxifloxacin should not be used as first-line therapy for complicated acute cystitis because it does not achieve sufficiently high urinary concentration. If gram-positive cocci are seen on Gram stain, enterococcus infection should be suspected, and ampicillin or amoxicillin should be added.

As antibiotic susceptibility data becomes available, antimicrobial coverage should be narrowed accordingly. The total treatment duration should be between 1 and 2 weeks. If the patient does not improve within 1 to 2 days, further evaluation should be performed to rule out an upper UTI or other complication (perinephric or renal abscess). Indwelling urinary catheters do not need to be routinely changed. However, patients with an indwelling urinary catheter who develop a UTI should have the catheter removed or replaced.

Cystitis in Patients with Diabetes

Patients with diabetes mellitus are at higher risk for having severe UTIs with complications. Pyelonephritis, perinephric abscess, renal abscess, and fungal infections occur with a greater frequency among patients with diabetes than in the general population. Asymptomatic bacteriuria in patients with diabetes should not be treated. The treatment of acute cystitis in patients with diabetes is discussed in the preceding section.

Emphysematous pyelonephritis

Emphysematous pyelonephritis is a condition that occurs almost exclusively in patients with diabetes and involves infection by gas-producing organisms. The history and physical findings are similar to those of acute pyelonephritis. There is a 6:1 female-to-male ratio, with an average age of 60. *E. coli* and *K. pneumoniae* are the two most common organisms identified (*E. coli* representing 69% of isolates, and *Klebsiella* 29%).

In addition to urinalysis, urine culture, and antibiotic sensitivity testing, radiologic imaging by CT should be performed to delineate the degree of infection and to help guide therapy. Antibiotic therapy with percutaneous catheter placement is the treatment of choice for patients with gas in the collecting system or in the renal parenchyma without involvement of the extrarenal area. Patients with extension of gas into the perinephric or pararenal spaces should be given antibiotics with percutaneous catheter placement if there is no renal dysfunction. Once renal dysfunction occurs, nephrectomy should be performed. Any patient that does not respond to antibiotics and percutaneous catheter drainage should also undergo nephrectomy.

Cystitis in Men

As in women, urethritis due to an STD should be ruled out. The first UTI should be treated with a 7-day course of a fluoroquinolone. Chronic prostatitis should be ruled out in men with recurrent UTIs.

Cystitis in Spinal Cord Injury Patients

Patients with spinal cord injury are at an increased risk of developing UTIs. They may present with atypical symptoms, such as urinary incontinence, diaphoresis, increased spasticity, autonomic hyperreflexia, or malaise. The most common pathogens are *E. coli*, enterococci and *Klebsiella*. A urinalysis, urine Gram stain, and culture should be performed before starting an empiric 7-day course of a fluoroquinolone. Presence of gram-positive cocci on the Gram stain should prompt addition of ampicillin or amoxicillin for enterococci coverage.

Uncomplicated Acute Pyelonephritis

As with uncomplicated acute cystitis, uncomplicated acute pyelonephritis is usually caused by *E. coli* and *S. saprophyticus*. Patients with nausea and vomiting precluding adequate oral intake, and those with severe disease or comorbidities that may result in an adverse outcome should be admitted for inpatient therapy.

A fluoroquinolone, such as ciprofloxacin or levofloxacin, should be used for empiric oral therapy of acute pyelonephritis. Further antibiotic choice should be tailored to the organism's antimicrobial susceptibility testing results. TMP, TMP-SMX, nitrofurantoin, sparfloxacin, and moxifloxacin should not be used as initial empiric therapy because of higher levels of resistance to TMP, TMP-SMX, and nitrofurantoin, and lower urinary concentrations of these fluoroquinolones. If Gram stain results demonstrate gram-positive cocci, amoxicillin should be added for enterococci coverage.

For empiric parenteral therapy of acute pyelonephritis, an intravenous fluoroquinolone (ciprofloxacin, levofloxacin, gatifloxacin), aminoglycoside, or broad-spectrum cephalosporin (ceftriaxone) may be used. Ampicillin should be added if there is a strong suspicion for enterococci.

Patients should be switched to oral antibiotics, as tolerated.

The standard treatment duration for uncomplicated acute pyelonephritis is 14 days. For mild to moderate cases, a 7-day treatment duration may be adequate, and for more severe cases, a 21-day course of antibiotics may be necessary.

Complicated Acute Pyelonephritis

Complicated acute pyelonephritis is associated with a wider range of pathogens, including *E. coli*, *Enterobacter*, *Pseudomonas*, *S. aureus*, and fungi.

A fluoroquinolone (ciprofloxacin, levofloxacin, gatifloxacin) should still be the initial empiric antimicrobial; further antibiotic selection should be guided by the organism's susceptibility results. Therapy should be continued for 14 days, with a repeat culture weeks after cessation of therapy to ascertain treatment success.

Renal Cortical Abscess (Renal Carbuncle)

Antibiotics targeting *S. aureus* should be instituted (nafcillin, oxacillin, or vancomycin for methicillin-resistant *S. aureus*) in addition to standard UTI therapy. Flank pain should improve within 24 hours, and fevers should improve within 6 days of starting therapy. Parenteral antibiotics should be continued for 2 weeks, and oral antibiotics should be given for an additional 2 to 4 weeks. If the patient does not respond within the initial 48 hours, percutaneous or surgical drainage should be performed.

Renal Corticomedullary Abscess

Antibiotic therapy should be the initial treatment of choice for renal corticomedullary abscesses confined to the renal parenchyma. Ciprofloxacin, third-generation cephalosporins (such as ceftriaxone, cefotaxime, or ceftazidime), or extended-spectrum beta-lactams (such as piperacillin or mezlocillin) may be used. Improvement is expected within 1 week. Intravenous antibiotics should be continued for 48 hours after resolution of fevers then oral therapy should be initiated for an additional 2 weeks.

Drainage procedures should be reserved for patients who do not respond to aggressive medical therapy.

Perinephric Abscess

Initial antibiotic therapy should include an anti-staphylococcal beta-lactam or cephalosporin with an aminoglycoside (oxacillin, nafcillin, cefazolin with tobramycin or gentamicin). Percutaneous drainage should be attempted and, if unsuccessful, surgical drainage is indicated. Ampicillin with an aminoglycoside should be initiated for enterococcal infection. Mezlocillin, piperacillin, cefoperazone, or ceftazidime should be used if *Pseudomonas* is isolated.

Asymptomatic Bacteriuria

Asymptomatic bacteriuria should be treated in pregnant patients, renal transplant patients, patients with nephrolithiasis, and prior to an invasive genitourinary procedure.

Treatment of asymptomatic bacteriuria is not indicated in elderly patients or patients with indwelling urinary catheters or intermittent urinary tract catheterization.

REFERENCES

Textbook Chapters

1. Chambers ST. Cystitis and Urethral Syndromes. In: Cohen J, Powderly WG, Berkley SF, et al. *Infectious Diseases*, 2nd ed. Philadelphia. Mosby, 2004. pp. 737–744.

2. Nicolle LE. Complicated Urinary Infection, Including Postsurgical and Catheter-related Infections. In: Cohen J, Powderly WG, Berkley SF, et al. *Infectious Diseases*, 2nd ed. Philadelphia. Mosby, 2004. pp. 763–770.

Guidelines

Warren JW, Abrutyn E, Hebel JR, et al. Guidelines from the Infectious Diseases Society of America. Guidelines for antimicrobial treatment of uncomplicated acute bacterial cystitis and acute pyelonephritis in women. *Clin Infect Dis*. 1999;29:745–758.

Review Articles

1. Hooton TM, Besser R, Foxman B, et al. Acute uncomplicated cystitis in an era of increasing antibiotic resistance: A proposed approach to empirical therapy. *Clin Infect Dis*. 2004;39:75–80.
2. Bergeron MG. Treatment of pyelonephritis in adults. *Med Clin North Am*. 1995;79:619–649.
3. Hooton TM, Stamm WE. Diagnosis and treatment of uncomplicated urinary tract infections. *Infect Dis Clin North Am*. 1997;11:551–582.
4. Dembry LM, Andriole VT. Renal and perirenal abscesses. *Infect Dis Clin North Am*. 1997;11:663–680.

Background and Epidemiology

Foxman B. Epidemiology of urinary tract infections: Incidence, mortality, and economic costs. *Am J Med*. 2002;113:Supplement 5S–13S.

Treatment

1. Gossius G, Vorland L. A randomized comparison of single-dose vs. three-day and ten-day therapy with trimethoprim-

sulfamethoxazole for acute cystitis in women. *Scand J Infect Dis*. 1984;16:373–379.

2. Inter-Nordic Urinary Tract Infection Study Group. Double-blind comparison of 3-day versus 7-day treatment with norfloxacin in symptomatic urinary tract infections. *Scand J Infect Dis*. 1988;20:619–624.

Miscellaneous

1. Hooton TM, Stamm WE. Diagnosis and treatment of uncomplicated urinary tract infections. *Infect Dis Clin North Am* 1997;11:551–582.

2. Warren JW, Abrutyn E, Hebel JR, et al. Guidelines from the Infectious Diseases Society of America. Guidelines for antimicrobial treatment of uncomplicated acute bacterial cystitis and acute pyelonephritis in women. *Clin Infect Dis*. 1999;29:745–758.

3. Chambers ST. Cystitis and Urethral Syndromes. In: Cohen J, Powderly WG, Berkley SF, et al. *Infectious Diseases*, 2nd ed. Philadelphia. Mosby, 2004. pp. 737–744.

4. Nicolle LE. Complicated urinary infection, including postsurgical and catheter-related infections. In: Cohen J, Powderly WG, Berkley SF, et al. *Infectious Diseases*, 2nd ed. Philadelphia. Mosby, 2004. pp. 763–770.

Pulmonary

CHAPTER 15

Acute Exacerbation of Chronic Obstructive Pulmonary Disease

KEY POINTS

1. Chronic obstructive pulmonary disease (COPD) refers to fixed airflow obstruction caused by chronic bronchitis (productive cough for at least 3 months of the year for at least 2 consecutive years) or emphysema (destruction of alveoli).

2. Tobacco smoking accounts for almost all cases of COPD.

3. Precipitants of COPD exacerbations include viral upper respiratory tract infections, bacterial infections (most commonly *Streptococcus pneumoniae*, *Haemophilus influenzae*, and *Moraxella catarrhalis*), pollution, heart failure, pulmonary embolism, and medications (beta-blockers, narcotics, sedatives).

4. There is no universally accepted definition of an acute exacerbation of COPD. The most commonly used definition is worsening dyspnea, an increase in sputum purulence, or an increase in sputum volume in a patient with COPD.

5. Symptoms and signs of COPD exacerbations include wheezing, distant breath sounds, tachypnea, tachycardia, accessory muscle use, cyanosis, agitation, confusion, and stupor.

6. Initial testing should include pulse oximetry, chest x-ray, and an electrocardiogram.

Other possible tests include arterial blood gas (if the patient's distress or somnolence raises concern for acute respiratory acidosis) and sputum Gram stain and culture (most appropriate for patients who fail to respond to empiric therapy).

7. Administer supplemental oxygen if there is hypoxemia. The goal oxygen saturation is 90% to 92% with a corresponding partial pressure of arterial oxygen of 60 to 65 mmHg. Higher oxygen saturations may cause hypercarbia by reducing the respiratory drive and promoting ventilation–perfusion mismatching.

8. Beta-agonists and anticholinergic agents are equally efficacious at improving airflow during a COPD exacerbation. Combination therapy is typically used in clinical practice, but does not appear to confer substantial benefit over monotherapy with either agent alone.

9. The role of aminophylline (methylxanthine bronchodilator) in the setting of a COPD exacerbation is controversial because this medication has uncertain efficacy and potential toxicity.

10. Systemic glucocorticoids improve FEV_1 and reduce treatment failure rates and length of hospitalization for a COPD exacerbation. The optimal dose, route, and duration of therapy are unknown.

11. Patients with a severe COPD exacerbation are the ones most likely to benefit from antibiotics, although the effect of antibiotics on the duration and severity of the exacerbation appears minimal. There are no definitive data regarding optimal duration of therapy.

12. Mucolytic agents and mechanical chest percussion are probably not beneficial in patients with a COPD exacerbation.

13. Many patients do not use metered-dose inhalers correctly. We recommend spacers to all patients, especially when inhaled glucocorticoids are prescribed.
14. Smoking cessation should be discussed. The pneumonia and influenza vaccines should be administered at the follow-up clinic visit, if applicable.

DEFINITIONS

Chronic bronchitis: Productive cough for at least 3 months of the year for at least 2 consecutive years. Other causes of chronic cough, such as gastroesophageal reflux disease, postnasal drip, and bronchiectasis, must be excluded.

Emphysema: Destruction of alveoli and abnormal distension of air spaces distal to the terminal bronchioles.

Chronic obstructive pulmonary disease (COPD): Fixed (not fully reversible), chronic airflow obstruction caused by chronic bronchitis or emphysema.

EPIDEMIOLOGY

COPD is a morbid, expensive, and lethal medical condition, affecting an estimated 16 million adults and accounting for 1.4 million emergency room visits in 1998. COPD was directly responsible for 1.9% of hospitalizations in 1998 and was a contributing cause of an additional 7% of hospitalizations during that year. Deaths related to COPD have been increasing steadily in the United States over the past 20 years, especially among women. COPD is now the fourth leading cause of death in the United States.

PATHOGENESIS

Tobacco smoking accounts for almost all cases of COPD. Cigarette smoke increases the number of neutrophils and macrophages in the airways. These cells release proteases (enzymes that degrade proteins), which destroy lung parenchyma in individuals who are unable to mount an adequate anti-protease response. As a result, mucus production is increased and airways become narrowed, lose their support structure, and develop increased collapsibility that leads to airway obstruction.

During an acute exacerbation of COPD, inflammation, bronchospasm, and mucus hypersecretion lead to airway narrowing, worsening ventilation–perfusion (V̇/Q̇) mismatching, and hypoxemia. The work of breathing increases to overcome the high airway resistance, but this leads to increased oxygen consumption by the respiratory muscles, which further lowers the oxygen content in venous blood.

PRECIPITANTS

COPD exacerbations become more frequent with increasing disease severity. An important trigger of these exacerbations is viral upper respiratory tract infections (especially rhinovirus), which cause airway inflammation and oxidative stress (Box 15-1). Although bacteria are often cultured from patients with an acute COPD exacerbation, it is unclear whether these organisms are pathogens or colonizers, because bacteria can also be cultured from many patients with stable COPD. The most common pathogenic bacteria are *Streptococcus pneumoniae*, *Haemophilus influenzae*, and *Moraxella catarrhalis*. COPD exacerbations are more common in the winter

Box 15-1. Causes of Chronic Obstructive Pulmonary Disease Exacerbations

Infection

Viruses

Rhinovirus (common cold)
Influenza
Parainfluenza
Coronavirus
Adenovirus
Respiratory syncytial virus
Chlamydia pneumoniae

Bacteria

Haemophilus influenza
Streptococcus pneumoniae
Moraxella catarrhalis
Staphylococcus aureus
Pseudomonas aeruginosa

Common Pollutants

Nitrogen dioxide
Particulates
Sulfur dioxide
Ozone

Medications

Sedatives and narcotics—reduce respiratory
     drive
Beta-blockers

Other

Congestive heart failure
Pulmonary embolism
Cold temperature—causes a small but significant
     reduction in lung function
Pneumothorax
No precipitant identified

Adapted with permission from Wedzicha JA. Exacerbations:
Etiology and pathophysiologic mechanisms. *Chest*
2002;121:136S–141S.

(upper respiratory tract infections are more common during these months, and cold temperatures to cause a small reduction in lung function). Exacerbations have also been linked to increasing environmental pollution, which is thought to increase susceptibility to viral respiratory infections.

Other precipitants of COPD exacerbations include heart failure, pulmonary embolism, and medications. Beta-blockers may cause bronchospasm, which can worsen ventilation–perfusion mismatch. Narcotics and sedatives may reduce the ventilatory drive, leading to hypercarbia, acidosis, and respiratory failure.

DIAGNOSIS

There is no universally accepted definition of an acute exacerbation of COPD. The most commonly used definition, which has been used most consistently in rigorous clinical trials, is any combination of the following three clinical findings in a patient with established COPD:

1. Worsening dyspnea
2. An increase in sputum purulence
3. An increase in sputum volume

Hypoxemia and hypercarbia are often present.

SIGNS

Mild COPD exacerbations may present with minimal signs, such as wheezing on auscultation. As the severity of COPD worsens, the breath sounds may be distant and there may be signs of hypoxemia including cyanosis, tachypnea, agitation, and tachycardia. Accessory muscle use may occur with the increased work of breathing. Inward abdominal motion with inspiration (abdominal paradox) is a sign of impending diaphragmatic muscle fatigue. With worsening respiratory failure, patients become increasingly hypercarbic and acidemic, which leads to confusion, stupor, and ultimately, apnea.

Laboratory Data

Initial laboratory testing should include:

1. **Pulse oximetry** to monitor the level of hypoxemia

2. **Chest x-ray**

   The classic findings of COPD include hyperinflated lungs, flattened diaphragms, and a narrowed and lengthened mediastinum. A chest x-ray should be obtained in all patients presenting with a COPD exacerbation because findings on radiography have been shown to change short-term management in as many as 20% of these patients, most of whom have new pulmonary infiltrates or evidence of heart failure.

3. **Arterial blood gas (ABG)**

   Most COPD exacerbations do not require ABG measurements. An ABG analysis is appropriate if the patient's distress or somnolence raises concern for acute respiratory acidosis, but the ABG should never delay intubation.

   Patients with stable COPD may have a chronic respiratory acidosis from long-standing carbon dioxide retention as a result of airway obstruction. ABG analysis in these patients shows an increased partial pressure of arterial carbon dioxide ($PaCO_2$) but normal arterial pH, because the kidneys buffer the acid by retaining bicarbonate. Patients with a superimposed acute respiratory acidosis will have a reduced arterial pH and higher $PaCO_2$ compared to their baseline measurements, because the kidneys are unable to buffer the acid resulting from acute carbon dioxide retention.

4. **Electrocardiogram (ECG)**

An admission ECG is recommended to rule out cardiac conditions, such as ischemia or acute myocardial infarction that may be contributing to the COPD exacerbation. Continuous cardiac monitoring is appropriate in patients with a moderate or severe COPD exacerbation, patients with a significant history of coronary artery disease, or patients with known cardiac arrhythmias, such as multifocal atrial tachycardia or atrial fibrillation.

5. **Sputum gram stain and culture**

White sputum may suggest a nonbacterial cause of the COPD exacerbation whereas green sputum may suggest a bacterial infection. However, sputum samples are notoriously unreliable, because they do not distinguish infection from colonization or oropharyngeal contamination. Therefore, sputum Gram stain and culture should be reserved for patients who do not respond to empiric therapy.

6. **Spirometry**

Spirometry is not recommended during a COPD exacerbation, because this technique does not provide a reliable measure of disease severity nor is it useful for guiding therapy.

ACUTE TREATMENT (Table 15-1, Fig. 15-1)

Supplemental Oxygen

Supplemental oxygen is appropriate if the COPD exacerbation is accompanied by hypoxemia. Oxygen saturation should be maintained between 90% and 92% with a corresponding partial pressure of arterial oxygen (PaO_2) of 60 to 65 mm Hg.

Table 15-1. Inpatient Management of an Acute Exacerbation of Chronic Obstructive Pulmonary Disease: Recommendations from Professional Societies

	British Thoracic Society	American College of Chest Physicians and American College of Physicians–American Society of Internal Medicine	European Respiratory Society	American Thoracic Society	Global Initiative for Chronic Obstructive Lung Disease (GOLD)
Date of statement	1997	2001	1995	1995	2001
Type of statement	Consensus	Evidenced-based review	Consensus	Consensus	Evidenced-based review
Diagnostic testing	Chest x-ray, arterial blood gas, complete blood count, electrolytes, ECG, sputum culture, FEV_1 or peak flow	Chest x-ray (spirometry is not recommended)	Chest x-ray, arterial blood gas, complete blood count, electrolytes, ECG, sputum gram stain and culture, FEV_1	Sputum culture if exacerbation is severe, if condition worsens despite antibiotics, or if patient is a nursing home resident	Chest x-ray, arterial blood gas, hematocrit, electrolytes, ECG, sputum culture

Continued

Table 15-1. Inpatient Management of an Acute Exacerbation of Chronic Obstructive Pulmonary Disease: Recommendations from Professional Societies—cont'd

	British Thoracic Society	American College of Chest Physicians and American College of Physicians–American Society of Internal Medicine	European Respiratory Society	American Thoracic Society	Global Initiative for Chronic Obstructive Lung Disease (GOLD)
Bronchodilators	Beta-agonists and anticholinergic agents. IV aminophylline if no response	Start with an anticholinergic agent. Add beta-agonist if maximal dose of the anticholinergic is inadequate. (Methylxanthines not recommended)	Beta agonists and anticholinergic agents. IV aminophylline in severe exacerbations	Start with beta-agonist ± anticholinergic agent. Add IV aminophylline if inadequate response	Start with beta-agonist. Add anticholinergic agent if prompt response not evident. Oral or IV methylxanthine in

Antibiotics	For moderate or severe exacerbations. Broader spectrum antibiotics if no response to first-line agents*	Optimal duration unclear	Inexpensive antibiotic for 7–14 days*	"Simple" antibiotic* for abnormal mucus. Broader spectrum antibiotic for severe exacerbations	severe exacerbations Antibiotic choice based on local sensitivity for S. pneumoniae, H. influenzae, M. catarrhalis
Glucocorticoids	Prednisone 30 mg daily for 7–14 days	Systemic for up to 2 weeks	Recommended, IV if severe exacerbation	Recommended, reassess use after 1–2 weeks	Oral or IV prednisolone daily for 10–14 days
Mucolytic drugs	Not recommended	Not recommended	Not recommended	Not recommended	Not discussed

Examples: amoxicillin, tetracycline, doxycycline.
ECG, electrocardiogram; FEV_1, forced expiratory volume in 1 second.

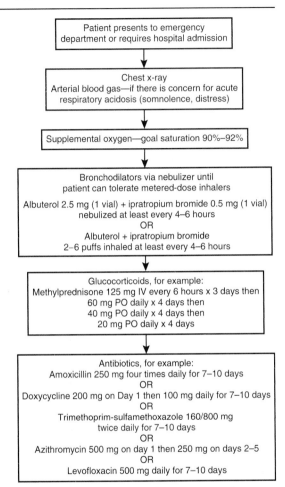

FIGURE 15–1. Initial treatment of an acute exacerbation of chronic obstructive pulmonary disease requiring hospitalization. Combination therapy is typically used in clinical practice but does not appear to confer substantial benefit over monotherapy with either agent alone.

These targets ensure near-maximal hemoglobin saturation. Higher oxygen saturations may cause hypercarbia by reducing the respiratory drive and promoting ventilation–perfusion mismatching.

There are several methods for delivering supplemental oxygen. Nasal cannula provides up to 6 L of oxygen per minute, although the actual percentage of oxygen inspired will depend on other factors, such as mouth-breathing. The concentration of oxygen in room air is 21%. As a general rule of thumb, for every 1 L of oxygen delivered per minute via nasal cannula, the inspired fraction of oxygen increases by 4%. The maximum oxygen delivery via nasal cannula is approximately 40%.

Non-rebreather face masks provide tighter control of inspired oxygen than nasal cannula. A partial non-rebreather mask has a reservoir that typically delivers 60% to 80% inspired oxygen. The reservoir bag is filled with oxygen that is emptied with inspiration. Exhalation fills the reservoir with the first portion of expired gas, which contains a high oxygen concentration derived from the dead space of the upper airway. A true non-rebreather mask contains two types of valves and can deliver close to 100% oxygen. One valve prevents exhaled gas from entering the reservoir bag. The second type of valve permits exhalation and prevents ambient air from entering the inhalation circuit.

Bronchodilators

Beta$_2$-agonists (albuterol) and anticholinergic agents (ipratropium bromide) are bronchodilators that are equally effective at improving airflow during a COPD exacerbation. These medications are commonly used together, although combination therapy does not appear to confer substantial benefit over monotherapy with either agent alone. Metered-dose inhalers (MDIs) and nebulizers appear to achieve equivalent bronchodilation, but MDIs cost less.

Aminophylline, a methylxanthine bronchodilator, has unclear efficacy and potential toxicity. Therefore, the role of this medication in the setting of a COPD exacerbation is unclear.

Glucocorticoids

Several good quality randomized trials have shown that systemic glucocorticoids are beneficial during an acute COPD exacerbation. Systemic glucocorticoids improve FEV_1 and reduce treatment failure rates and length of hospitalization. The shortest useful duration of therapy is unknown, but there appears to be no additional advantage when glucocorticoids are given for more than 2 weeks. Oral and parenteral glucocorticoids appear to have similar efficacy. Improved outcomes have been demonstrated with doses ranging from 40 mg of oral prednisone daily in outpatient and emergency department settings to 125 mg of intravenous methylprednisone every 6 hours for 3 days, followed by 60 mg of oral prednisone daily for 4 days and then a gradual tapering of the dose with discontinuation on Day 15 in hospitalized patients. However, the optimal dose, route, and duration of therapy are unknown and vary among physicians and patients.

Hyperglycemia is an important side effect of short-term glucocorticoid treatment. Patients with frequent exacerbations may also experience bone loss from repeated courses of glucocorticoids. Infection is unlikely with short-term treatment.

Antibiotics

Bacterial infections may contribute to acute COPD exacerbations. Several randomized trials have shown that patients with severe COPD exacerbations are the most likely to benefit from antibiotics, although the effect of antibiotics on the duration and severity of the exacerbation appears minimal. Trials have most commonly prescribed tetracyclines, amoxicillin, or trimethoprim-sulfamethoxazole for 3 to 14 days to cover the three most common causal pathogens: *S. pneumoniae, M. catarrhalis,* and *H. influenzae*. Nowadays, more broad-spectrum antibiotics, such as levofloxacin, are commonly used in clinical practice because of emerging antibiotic resistance (especially among *S. pneumoniae*). The superiority of these newer, broader-spectrum antibiotics has not been established. There are also no definitive data regarding optimal duration of therapy, so most physicians prescribe antibiotics for 5 to 10 days.

Mucolytic Agents

Several studies have shown no beneficial effects of mucolytic agents or mechanical chest percussion in patients with a COPD exacerbation.

Noninvasive Positive-Pressure Ventilation (NPPV)

NPPV unloads fatigued ventilatory muscles and reduces the rates of intubation, in-hospital mortality, and duration of hospitalization. NPPV is appropriate for the COPD patient with acute respiratory acidosis, and worsening dyspnea and oxygenation, provided the patient is cooperative, hemodynamically stable, does not have excessive secretions, and is able to protect the airway. Patients who cannot tolerate NPPV and who have worsening oxygenation or acidemia should be intubated.

IS THE PATIENT READY FOR HOSPITAL DISCHARGE?

Patients are ready for hospital discharge when significant clinical improvement has occurred. A useful question to ask the patient is whether the clinical status is close to baseline. Bronchospasm should be minimal or absent, and oxygen saturation with ambulation should not fall below 88%. Patients with persistent hypoxemia

Box 15-2. Basic Use of a Metered-Dose Inhaler (MDI) with a Spacer

The patient should:

- Shake the inhaler and attach it to the spacer.
- Breath out, then form a seal around the mouthpiece of the spacer.
- Depress the canister, then breathe in slowly through the mouth.
- Hold the breath for 10 seconds or as long as possible.
- Wait a minute or so, then repeat the above steps, if applicable.
- Rinse the mouth after using an inhaled glucocorticoid to reduce the risk of oral candidiasis.

despite resolution of symptoms should be discharged with supplemental oxygen via nasal cannula.

Many patients do not use MDIs correctly. Patients may experience difficulty coordinating inhalation with the release of medication from the canister. Therefore, we recommend spacers to all patients, especially when inhaled glucocorticoids are prescribed (Box 15-2).

At the followup clinic visit, smoking cessation should be discussed and the conjugated pneumococcal vaccine and influenza vaccines should be administered (if the patient is due for these vaccines). Spirometry before and after a several-week trial of inhaled glucocorticoids should be used to assess whether the patient's COPD has a reversible component (i.e., whether the patient will benefit from long-term glucocorticoids).

REFERENCES

Review Articles and Position Papers

1. Palm KH, Decker WW. Acute exacerbations of chronic obstructive pulmonary disease. *Emerg Med Clin North Am.* 2003;21:331–352.
2. Stoller JK. Acute exacerbations of chronic obstructive pulmonary disease. *N Engl J Med.* 2002;346:988–994.
3. Bach PB, Brown C, Gelfand SE, McCrory DC. Management of acute exacerbations of chronic obstructive pulmonary disease: A summary and appraisal of published evidence. *Ann Intern Med.* 2001;134:600–620.

Epidemiology

Mannino DM. COPD: Epidemiology, prevalence, morbidity and mortality, and disease heterogeneity. *Chest* 2002;121:121S–126S.

Pathogenesis of Exacerbations

Wedzicha JA. Exacerbations: Etiology and pathophysiologic mechanisms. *Chest* 2002; 121:136S–141S.

Treatment

1. Irwin RS, Madison JM. Systemic corticosteroids for acute exacerbations of chronic obstructive pulmonary disease. *N Engl J Med.* 2003;348:2679–2681.
2. Snow V, Lascher S, Mottur-Pilson C. The evidence base for management of acute exacerbations of COPD: Clinical practice guideline. *Chest* 2001;119:1185–1189.
3. Singh JM, Palda VA, Stanbrook MB, Chapman KR. Corticosteroid therapy for patients with acute exacerbation of chronic obstructive pulmonary disease: A systematic review. *Arch Intern Med.* 2002;162:2527–2536.

4. Saint S, Bent S, Vittinghoff E, Grady D. Antibiotics in chronic obstructive pulmonary disease exacerbations: A meta-analysis. *JAMA* 1995;273:957–960.

5. Callahan CM, Dittus RS, Katz BP. Oral corticosteroid therapy for patients with stable chronic obstructive pulmonary disease: A meta-analysis. *Ann Intern Med*. 1991;114:216–2236.

6. Niewoehner DE, Erbland ML, Deupree RH, Collins D, et al. Effect of systemic glucocorticoids on exacerbations of chronic obstructive pulmonary disease. Department of Veterans Affairs Cooperative Study Group. *N Engl J Med*. 1999;340:1941–1947.

CHAPTER 16

Acute Asthma

KEY POINTS

1. Asthma is a chronic inflammatory respiratory disease that is increasing in prevalence and accounts for $6 billion in health care costs annually.
2. The pathogenesis of asthma involves bronchoconstriction, airway edema, mucus plug formation, and airway remodeling.
3. Important asthma triggers include environmental factors (tobacco smoke, perfumes, animal dander, dust mites, and pollen), infections (respiratory infections, sinusitis), and medications (NSAIDs and beta blockers).
4. Regular peak expiratory flow rate monitoring is indicated in patients with moderate or severe asthma. A baseline "personal best" should be established, and an action plan developed for differing percentages of the personal best.
5. The diagnosis of asthma rests on the presence of symptoms of airways obstruction, demonstration of at least partial reversibility, and exclusion of alternate diagnoses.
6. Inpatient treatment of acute asthma relies on the use of systemic corticosteroids, inhaled bronchodilators, oxygen, and, if necessary, intubation with mechanical ventilation for patients with impending or actual respiratory failure.
7. Use of methylxanthines, mucolytics, or sedatives is not indicated for the management of acute asthma.

DEFINITION

Asthma is defined by the National Asthma Education and Prevention Program, Expert Panel Report 2 (EPR2), as a chronic inflammatory disorder of the airways.

Severe persistent asthma causes continuous symptoms with frequent exacerbations and physical activity limitations. Patients frequently have nocturnal symptoms. The forced expiratory volume in 1 second (FEV_1) or peak expiratory flow rate (PEFR) is < 60% of predicted, and the PEFR variability is greater than 30%.

Moderate persistent asthma is associated with daily symptoms (despite daily use of inhaled short-acting beta-2 agonists) with > 2 exacerbations weekly, causing limitations in activity. Patients have more than 1 episode of nocturnal symptoms weekly. FEV_1 or PEFR is between 60% and 80% of predicted, with a PEFR variability greater than 30%.

Mild persistent asthma induces symptoms more than twice a week, but less than every day, with exacerbations causing activity limitations. Nocturnal symptoms occur more than twice a month. FEV_1 or PEFR is > 80% of predicted, and the PEFR variability is between 20% and 30%.

Mild intermittent asthma causes symptoms less than twice a week, with normal PEFR between exacerbations. Nocturnal symptoms occur less than twice a month, and the FEV_1 or PEFR is > 80% of predicted. The PEFR variability is less than 30%.

In this chapter, we focus on inpatient management of acute asthma.

EPIDEMIOLOGY

Asthma affects approximately 15 million persons in the United States, accounts for almost 500,000 hospitalizations per year, and causes approximately 5000 deaths annually. The prevalence of asthma is increasing worldwide. Hospitalization rates for acute asthma are highest among children and African Americans. African Americans between 15 and 24 years of age have the highest mortality rate from asthma.

Acute asthma is the 11th most frequent condition seen in the emergency department, representing up to 12% of total cases. Approximately, 30% of patients with acute asthma are ultimately hospitalized, and 4% to 7% of admitted patients required care in the intensive care unit.

In terms of health care expenditures, the United States spends $6 billion on asthma care; hospital-based care (emergency department visits and admissions) accounts for one half those costs. Better outpatient management will likely result in the greatest savings in health care costs.

Pathogenesis

Asthma is a disorder involving chronic airways inflammation, resulting in airflow obstruction due to:

- Bronchoconstriction
  - May be caused by IgE-dependent release of histamine, leukotrienes, tryptase, and prostaglandins from mast cells
  - Bronchoconstriction caused by NSAIDs, exercise, or cold air is not IgE mediated.
- Airway edema
  - Inflammatory mediators cause increased vascular permeability, resulting in mucosal swelling and airway narrowing
- Formation of mucus plugs
- Remodeling of the airways
  - Alterations in the extracellular matrix and fibrosis below the basement membrane
  - This component may result in airway obstruction that is only partially reversible

These inflammatory changes, along with airway hyperresponsiveness, cause airflow obstruction and result in symptoms of dyspnea, wheezing, and cough. Airway hyperresponsiveness can be induced by administration of methacholine or histamine. Atopy is the most important identifiable risk factor for the development of asthma.

Numerous potential triggers of airway inflammation have been identified and include respiratory infections, environmental allergens, tobacco smoke, NSAIDs, exercise, cold air, and gastroesophageal reflux disease.

CLINICAL FEATURES

History

The history should focus on confirming the diagnosis of asthma, identifying potential symptom triggers, and determining disease severity.

Symptoms of dyspnea, cough, wheezing, and chest tightness are consistent with asthma. Studies have found that patients with asthma present with dyspnea in 29%, cough in 24%, and wheezing in 35% of cases. The symptoms tend to worsen at night. Patients may also have intermittent symptoms that occur with certain seasons or times of day.

Symptom pattern and duration should be established. Patients should be asked about age at initial diagnosis, frequency of symptoms, medication use, corticosteroid requirements, prior hospitalizations and any previous intubations, comorbid conditions, and overall disease course (improving or worsening since diagnosis).

Precipitating factors that could either trigger or worsen an asthma attack should be explored:

- Infectious—e.g., viral respiratory infections, sinusitis

- Environmental triggers—tobacco smoke, pollen, mold, dust mites, cockroaches, pets, cold air, occupational exposures, strong odors, such as perfume
- Medications—NSAIDs, aspirin, beta-blockers
- Food exposures—e.g., sulfites, preservatives
- Miscellaneous—exercise, menses, pregnancy, thyroid disease, and gastroesophageal reflux disease

Known triggers can be avoided, which may decrease the number of acute asthma episodes.

Determination of the severity of asthma is important. The most specific risk for development of fatal asthma is repeated admissions for asthma flares, particularly if the admissions require mechanical ventilation. Patients who have required mechanical ventilation have a 10% mortality rate at 1 year and a 23% mortality at 6 years. Other markers of severity are:

- Use of systemic glucocorticoids
- History of medical non-compliance
- Older age
- Use of tobacco
- History of atopy or aspirin-induced asthma

Physical Examination

Physical examination may reveal expiratory wheezing, hyperexpansion of the thorax, or a prolonged expiratory phase. In addition, signs of atopy, such as eczema, atopic dermatitis, nasal discharge or mucosal edema, or nasal polyps may be seen. Evidence of potential triggers, such as respiratory infections, should be sought.

Accessory muscle use, intercostal retractions, or pulsus paradoxus (fall in systolic blood pressure greater than 10 mmHg with inspiration) are indicators of potential respiratory distress.

Peak Expiratory Flow Rate (PEFR)

PEFR monitoring is a simple and cost-effective means of determining the degree of airways obstruction. PEFR is a tool for monitoring patients with asthma, but it should not be used for the diagnosis of asthma. Patients with moderate or severe asthma should be instructed in the use of PEFR and have a peak flow meter accessible for self-monitoring.

Patients should establish a baseline "personal best" PEFR. At a time when asthma symptoms are well-controlled, readings should be obtained at least twice daily over a 2- to 3-week period, with one reading when the patient wakes up and another between noon and 2:00 PM. Readings should also be obtained pre– and post–beta-2 agonist use.

PEFR zones are defined by the EPR2 as follows:

- Green Zone: > 80% of personal best peak flow. These readings represent good asthma control, and patients should continue taking their medications without change.
- Yellow Zone: > 50%, but < 80% of personal best peak flow. Patients with readings in this range should exercise caution. A short-acting inhaled beta-2 agonist should be taken immediately, and the patient should contact the physician regarding any potential changes to the asthma regimen.
- Red Zone: < 50% of personal best peak flow. Patients should be on the alert, take their short-acting inhaled beta-2 agonist, and contact their physician or the emergency department immediately. Patients may also go to their nearest emergency room.

Aside from their use in monitoring acute exacerbations of asthma, measurement of PEFR is also useful in assessing patient response to changes in their asthma regimen.

DIAGNOSIS

According to EPR2, the diagnosis of asthma relies on demonstrating:

- Presence of symptoms of episodic airway obstruction
- At least partial reversibility of airflow obstruction
- Exclusion of other alternative diagnoses

Spirometry

Spirometry (FEV_1, forced vital capacity [FVC], and FEV_1/FVC) should be performed in a non-acute setting before and after bronchodilator administration. An FEV_1 less than 80% of predicted, and an FEV_1/FVC ratio of less than 65% are consistent with airway obstruction. Reversibility is present if there is at least a 12% and 200 mL increase in the FEV_1. If reversibility is not demonstrated initially, a trial of corticosteroids may be administered, and the test repeated in 2 to 3 weeks.

Spirometry with methacholine (or histamine) challenge may be performed in patients with atypical presentations of asthma, such as isolated cough, or exercise-induced symptoms. Spirometry is measured at baseline and after nebulized saline. If there is no change in the FEV_1, methacholine is administered in increasing doses until either a 20% decrease in FEV_1 is noted (positive test) or the highest concentration of methacholine is reached (negative test). Although a positive test is not specific for asthma, a negative test rules out asthma with approximately 95% certainty.

Patients with a history highly suggestive of asthma but negative spirometry testing should be evaluated with either serial spirometry (due to intermittent or diurnal symptoms) or provocation testing.

Spirometry should be repeated every 1 to 2 years to establish new baselines as the disease progresses.

Additional Tests

Lung volumes and diffusion capacity may be measured to help distinguish chronic obstructive pulmonary disease from asthma; patients with asthma should have normal baseline lung function between episodes. A chest x-ray may be performed to exclude other diagnoses, such as allergic bronchopulmonary aspergillosis or pulmonary infiltrates with eosinophilia.

Allergy testing may be helpful in identifying potential asthma triggers so that they may be minimized, avoided, or eliminated. Common allergens that are assessed are dust mites, animal dander, cockroach antigen, pollen, and mold.

Patients with atopy may have eosinophilia, as will patients with parasitic infections causing Loeffler's syndrome. Evaluation for gastroesophageal reflux disease may also be indicated.

TREATMENT

Overview

Long-term medications (corticosteroids, long-acting beta-2 agonists, leukotriene-modifying agents) are used daily to facilitate prevention or control of asthma flares. Quick-relief medications are used to rapidly relieve airflow obstruction, and include short-acting beta-2 agonists, anticholinergics, and systemic corticosteroids (although the benefits of corticosteroids are not evident for at least 4 hours after administration).

Particular caution should be taken in the management of patients with risk factors for fatal asthma (from EPR2):

- History of intubation(s) for asthma exacerbations or admission to the intensive care unit

- History of severe and sudden asthma exacerbations
- Two or more hospitalizations or three or more emergency department visits for asthma exacerbations within the last year
- Asthma exacerbation requiring hospitalization or emergency room care within the last month
- Use of more than two short-acting beta-2 agonist metered dose inhalers per month
- Current or recent use of systemic corticosteroids
- Other medical or psychiatric comorbidities
- Illicit drug use
- Low socioeconomic status

MANAGEMENT IN AN EMERGENCY DEPARTMENT OR URGENT CARE SETTING

Initial Assessment and Therapy (Box 16-1)

The history and physical examination should be targeted to potential triggers, markers of severity, and exclusion of alternate diagnoses, as has been described. Measurement of PEFR prior to the initiation of therapy provides a baseline for comparison. Pulse oximetry should be obtained.

Arterial blood gas should be obtained in patients with a PEFR or FEV_1 less than 30% of predicted. In patients with an asthma exacerbation, the pCO_2 should be less than 40 mm Hg because of hyperventilation. Therefore, a pCO_2 near normal is concerning for impending respiratory failure. A complete blood count may be helpful to assess for infection as a potential trigger. Chest x-ray should be obtained in patients with a suspected cardiopulmonary complication, such as pneumothorax, pneumonia, or congestive heart failure. Patients with cardiac risk factors may warrant an electrocardiogram.

Supplemental oxygen should be administered to maintain saturation > 90% (> 95% in pregnant patients and those with cardiac comorbidities). Short-acting beta-2 agonists should be administered, either continuously or every 20 minutes for 1 hour.

Patients with Impending or Actual Respiratory Arrest

Patients with a $pCO_2 > 42$ mm Hg, decreased mental alertness, or signs of respiratory fatigue are at risk for respiratory arrest, and should be admitted to the intensive care unit intubated and provided with mechanical ventilation with 100% oxygen. Intravenous corticosteroids, such as methylprednisolone, 120 to 180 mg total dose per day, given in three to four divided doses, should be started. Nebulized short-acting beta-2 agonists and anticholinergics should be administered.

Patients with Severe Asthma Exacerbation (PEFR or FEV_1 < 50%)

Patients with risk factors for fatal asthma or physical examination demonstrating accessory muscle use or intercostal retractions fall into the severe asthma exacerbation category.

Supplemental oxygen and an oral systemic corticosteroid (such as prednisone 60 mg orally) should be administered. A short-acting beta-2 agonist with an anticholinergic should be administered either continuously or every 20 minutes for 1 hour.

Patients with Moderate Exacerbation (PEFR or FEV_1 > 50%)

Supplemental oxygen should be given and a short-acting beta-2 agonist with an anticholinergic should be administered either continuously or every 20 minutes for 1 hour. Oral systemic corticosteroids (such as prednisone 60 mg orally) should be given if the patient does not have a complete response to the initial trial of bronchodilator therapy.

Reevaluation and Further Therapy

Patients with moderate or severe asthma should be reevaluated after the initial therapy described previously. Patients with PEFR or FEV_1 between 50% and 80% who respond to initial therapy should be maintained on systemic corticosteroids. Inhaled short-acting beta-2 agonists should be administered every 60 minutes. This treatment regimen should be continued for 1 to 3 hours with close monitoring.

High-risk patients with PEFR or FEV_1 < 50% should be continued on systemic corticosteroids and continuous inhaled short-acting beta-2 agonists with an anticholinergic agent. Close monitoring for impending respiratory failure is essential.

Patients that are able to achieve and maintain a PEFR or FEV_1 > 70% for longer than 1 hour may be discharged home with continued systemic corticosteroids, inhaled short-acting beta-2 agonists, close outpatient follow-up, and a definitive action plan for repeat exacerbations.

Incomplete responders to initial therapy with a PEFR or FEV_1 > 50% and < 70% and moderate signs and symptoms should be continued on oral or intravenous systemic corticosteroids and inhaled short-acting beta-2 agonists with an anticholinergic agent. Admission to a hospital ward should be considered for high-risk patients and patients with inconsistent or unreliable outpatient follow-up. Lower-risk patients with excellent medication compliance and outpatient care may be considered for discharge.

Patients failing to respond to initial treatment, with a PEFR or FEV_1 < 50%, should be admitted to the intensive care unit. If the patient continues to deteriorate, intubation with mechanical ventilation may be necessary. Intravenous corticosteroids, inhaled short-acting beta-2 agonists with an anticholinergic agent, and oxygen should be administered. Patients who improve may eventually be transferred to a hospital ward for further therapy.

Patients admitted to a hospital ward may be treated with systemic corticosteroids and inhaled short-acting beta-2 agonists with an anticholinergic agent (see Box 16–1 for routine dosages). Management of mechanical ventilation in patients with acute asthma is beyond the scope of this chapter.

Box 16-1. Medication Dosages for the Treatment of Acute Asthma

Corticosteroids

- Prednisone 120–180 mg daily in three to four divided doses for up to 2 days. Then taper to 60–80 mg daily when the peak expiratory flow rate (PEFR) improves to greater than 70% of predicted or personal best. Equivalent dosages of other corticosteroids may be used.
- Prednisone 40–60 mg daily in two divided doses for 3–10 days may be used for outpatient management of acute asthma exacerbations.

Inhaled short-acting beta$_2$ agonists

- Albuterol nebulized solution: 2.5–5 mg every 20 min for three doses, then every 1–4 hr as needed. For severe exacerbations, use the 5 mg dosing. May also use 10–15 mg continuous nebulized solution.
- Albuterol metered dose inhaler (MDI) (90 µg/puff): four to eight puffs every 20 min for up to 4 hr, then every 1–4 hr as needed.

Anticholinergic agents

- Ipratropium bromide nebulized solution: 0.5 mg every 30 min for three doses, then every 2–4 hr as needed. May be combined with albuterol nebulized solution.
- Ipratropium bromide MDI (18 µg/puff): four to eight puffs as needed.

Medications to avoid

- Methylxanthines, mucolytics, and sedatives are not recommended for treatment of acute asthma exacerbation.
- Routine use of antibiotics in patients without evidence of infection (e.g., fevers, purulent sputum) is not generally recommended.

Hospital Discharge

At the time of discharge, patients should be converted to oral and inhaled medications. Intravenous corticosteroids should be converted to their oral or inhaled equivalents (whichever is appropriate), and bronchodilators should preferably be administered via an MDI.

Patients should be instructed on proper MDI and PEFR meter usage and understand the importance of the "green, yellow, and red" zones (see preceding text). Beta-2 agonists delivered through nebulizers or MDI are equally efficacious when MDIs are properly used. Please see Chapter 15 for a discussion on proper MDI technique.

Close follow-up with a primary care provider and, if necessary, referral to a pulmonologist should be facilitated.

REFERENCES

Guidelines

1. National Asthma Education and Prevention Program Expert Panel Report 2. Guidelines for the Diagnosis and Management of Asthma. U.S. Department of Health and Human Services, National Institutes of Health, Bethesda, 1997.

2. National Asthma Education and Prevention Program Expert Panel Report: Guidelines for the Diagnosis and Management of Asthma. Update on Selected Topics 2002. *J Allergy Clin Immunol*. 2002;110:S141.

Review Articles

1. Wenzel SE, Fahy JV, Irvin C, et al. American Thoracic Society. Proceedings of the ATS Workshop on Refractory Asthma. *Am J Resp Crit Care Med*. 2000;162:2341–2351.
2. Nadel JA, Busse WW. Asthma. *Am J Resp Crit Care Med*. 1998;157:S130–S138.
3. Rodrigo GJ, Rodrigo C, Hall JB. Acute asthma in adults—a review. *Chest* 2004;125:1081–1102.
4. Busse WW, Lemanske Jr RF. Asthma. *N Engl J Med*. 2001;344:350–362.

Treatment

1. Donohue JF. Therapeutic responses in asthma and COPD—bronchodilators. *Chest* 2004;126:125S–137S.
2. Larj MJ, Bleeker ER. Therapeutic responses in asthma and COPD—corticosteroids. *Chest* 2004;126:138S–149S.
3. Ho AM, Lee A, Karmakar MK, et al. Heliox vs air–oxygen mixtures for the treatment of patients with acute asthma. *Chest* 2003;123:882–890.
4. Rodrigo GJ, Rodrigo C, Pollack CV, et al. use of helium–oxygen mixtures in the treatment of acute asthma. *Chest* 2003;123:891–896.

Renal

Acute Renal Failure

1. Acute renal failure (ARF) refers to an abrupt decline in renal function.
2. There is no universally accepted laboratory definition of ARF.
3. Pre-renal ARF occurs when decreased renal perfusion leads to a reduction in the glomerular filtration rate.
4. Intrinsic ARF occurs when there is injury to the renal glomeruli, tubules, interstitium, or vessels. Acute tubular necrosis is the most common cause of intrinsic ARF.
5. Post-renal ARF results from obstruction of the urinary collecting system.
6. Most patients with ARF are asymptomatic and are diagnosed based on laboratory data.
7. Initial testing in patients with ARF should include urinalysis and measurement of electrolytes, urine output, serum calcium, phosphate, and magnesium. Depending on the clinical circumstances, other tests may include renal ultrasonography, complete blood count, coagulation panel, urine eosinophils, creatine phosphokinase, and calculation of the fractional excretion of sodium (FE_{Na}).
8. The serum creatinine concentration does not accurately reflect the glomerular filtration rate in the nonsteady state of ARF.

9. The blood urea nitrogen-to-creatinine ratio is usually >20:1 in prerenal disease.

10. In oliguric patients, $FE_{Na} < 1\%$ usually suggests prerenal ARF whereas $FE_{Na} > 2\%$ usually suggests intrinsic renal disease.

11. The approach to renal failure should include determination of (a) chronicity, (b) patient comorbidities, (c) whether there has been a recent vascular intervention, (d) whether the patient has received intravenous contrast or other nephrotoxic medications, and (e) volume status.

12. General management principles of ARF include (a) institution of a "renal" diet, (b) adjusting dosages of all medications metabolized or excreted by the kidneys, (c) discontinuing nephrotoxins or substituting non-nephrotoxic alternatives (if possible), (d) monitoring fluid status, and (e) monitoring and treating complications of ARF (such as hyperkalemia, hyponatremia, and hyperphosphatemia).

13. Prompt treatment of renal obstruction can lead to complete recovery of renal function. Post-obstructive diuresis (4–20 L/day), which sometimes occurs following correction of bilateral urinary obstruction, can lead to hypovolemia, hypokalemia, and hypomagnesemia.

14. Diuretics do not reduce mortality or the need for dialysis in ARF patients.

15. Low-dose intravenous dopamine (1–3 µg/kg/min) does not reduce mortality or promote recovery of renal function in patients with ARF.

DEFINITIONS

Acute renal failure (ARF): Abrupt decline in renal function leading to retained nitrogenous and non-nitrogenous waste products. Sufficiently severe ARF will cause metabolic derangements including hyponatremia, hyperkalemia, hyperphosphatemia, metabolic acidosis, and fluid retention. There is no universally accepted laboratory definition of ARF. One definition is an increase in serum creatinine of at least 0.5 mg/dL within 2 weeks (or a creatinine increase of at least 20% if the baseline creatinine is above 2.5 mg/dL).

Oliguria: Urine output < 400 mL/day. Oliguria generally implies more severe renal injury than non-oliguria. However, urine output can be normal in patients with severe ARF.

Anuria: Urine output < 100 mL/day.

EPIDEMIOLOGY

The incidence of ARF varies according to the definition used and the population studied. The incidence of hospital-acquired ARF is close to 5% although up to 20% of critically ill patients develop an episode of ARF during their illness.

PATHOPHYSIOLOGY

The pathophysiology of ARF is easiest to conceptualize when patients are classified according to the site of the abnormality (Box 17-1).

Pre-Renal

Pre-renal ARF develops when decreased renal perfusion leads to a reduction in the glomerular filtration rate (GFR). This can occur in patients with hypovolemia or reduced effective circulating volume (such as heart failure, cirrhosis, or the

Box 17-1. Causes of Acute Renal Failure

Pre-Renal

Hypovolemia or reduced effective circulating blood volume

Hypotension, including sepsis, anesthesia, medication-induced

Drugs—Nonsteroidal anti-inflammatory drugs, angiotensin-converting enzyme inhibitors

Large vessel thrombosis, embolus, or dissection

Hepatorenal syndrome

Intrarenal

Small vessel

Atheroembolism, malignant hypertension, scleroderma, TTP/HUS, DIC

Glomerulus

Glomerulonephritis

Vasculitis

Tubules

Acute tubular necrosis

Ischemic—hypovolemia, hypotension, sepsis

Toxic—IV contrast, aminoglycosides, amphotericin B, cisplatin, heme-pigments

Obstruction—uric acid, calcium oxalate, acyclovir, indinavir, light chains

Interstitium

Acute interstitial nephritis

Infiltration—lymphoma, sarcoidosis

Bilateral pyelonephritis

Post-Renal

Ureteral

Tumors, calculi, sloughed papillae, retroperitoneal fibrosis, lymphadenopathy

Bladder neck

Tumors, calculi, prostatic hypertrophy or carcinoma, neurogenic

Urethral

Strictures, tumors, obstructed indwelling
   catheters

nephrotic syndrome) and almost always presents
with oliguria. The kidneys attempt to compensate
for the reduced blood flow and maintain GFR by
dilating afferent arterioles (via prostaglandins)
and constricting efferent arterioles (via angiotensin II). Renal failure develops when these compensatory mechanisms are inadequate or impaired
as sometimes occurs in hypovolemic patients who
are simultaneously receiving a nonsteroidal anti-
inflammatory drug (which reduces prostaglandin
production) and an angiotensin-converting enzyme
inhibitor (which reduces formation of angiotensin
II). Initially, the integrity of the renal parenchyma
is preserved in all cases of prerenal disease. However, persistent, uncorrected renal hypoperfusion
will ultimately lead to ischemic injury.

Intrinsic

Intrinsic ARF occurs when there is injury to the
renal glomeruli, tubules, interstitium, or vessels.
The most common cause of intrinsic ARF is acute
tubular necrosis (ATN), which develops when there
is ischemic or toxic injury to the kidney, as can occur
with sepsis, aminoglycoside antibiotics, some che-
motherapies, and intravenous radiocontrast agents.
Pre-renal ARF of sufficient severity and duration
will cause ischemic ATN. Other causes of intrinsic
ARF include glomerulonephritis, allergic interstitial
nephritis (AIN), rhabdomyolysis, atheroembolic
disease, and multiple myeloma light-chain proteins.

The mechanisms of rhabdomyolysis-induced ARF include (1) renal vasoconstriction, (2) myoglobin precipitation leading to cast formation and tubular obstruction, and (3) ischemic injury (myoglobin degradation causes free radical production and lipid peroxidation).

Atheroembolic disease (cholesterol embolism) involving the renal arteries, arterioles, and glomerular capillaries can cause sudden ARF or a stepwise decline in renal function over several months. Atheroembolic disease occurs spontaneously, or as a result of atheromatous plaque disruption during an intravascular intervention (such as injury to the aorta during coronary angioplasty), or when administration of anticoagulants prevents healing of an eroded plaque.

Intravenous contrast agents cause direct tubular epithelial cell toxicity and renal medullary ischemia. Risk factors for contrast nephropathy include diabetes mellitus, baseline renal disease, volume depletion, and concurrent nephrotoxic drugs (Box 17–2).

Post-Renal

Post-renal ARF results from obstruction of the urinary collecting system and accounts for approximately 5% of hospital-acquired ARF.

Box 17-2. Risk Factors for Radiocontrast-Induced Nephrotoxicity

Advanced age
Renal insufficiency
Decreased absolute and effective circulatory volume
Diabetes mellitus
Multiple myeloma
Co-administration of other nephrotoxic agents

Reproduced with permission from Palmer BF, Henrich WL. Toxic nephropathy. In: Brenner BM, editor. *Brenner and Rector's The Kidney*, 7th ed. Philadelphia: Saunders; 2004. p. 1630.

SYMPTOMS AND SIGNS

Most patients with ARF are asymptomatic and are diagnosed based on laboratory data. Patients with prerenal ARF may have a history of vomiting, diarrhea, hypotension, hemorrhage, or excessive diuresis. On physical examination, these patients may have tachycardia, hypotension, postural signs, and dry mucus membranes. Patients with intrinsic ARF may have received nephrotoxic medications or intravenous contrast or may have features of systemic disease, such as rhabdomyolysis or vasculitis. Livedo reticularis (purplish rash over the lower extremities and abdominal wall) suggests atheroembolic disease, which can also present with constitutional symptoms and multisystem involvement. Patients with postrenal ARF may have benign prostatic hypertrophy or abdominal symptoms originating from a tumor. On physical examination, these patients may have a distended bladder, enlarged prostate, or a palpable abdominal mass.

Patients with sufficiently severe ARF, regardless of the cause, may have signs of uremia, including lethargy, nausea, confusion, volume overload, and electrolyte abnormalities (such as hyponatremia and hyperkalemia).

Laboratory Data

Initial laboratory testing for patients with ARF should include the following (obtaining some of these tests may depend upon the clinical circumstances):

1. Electrolytes including blood urea nitrogen and creatinine
2. Urinalysis and urine sediment
3. Accurate assessment of urine output—may require bladder catheterization if the patient is unable to accurately collect urine (dementia or urinary incontinence)

4. Urinary sodium and creatinine for calculation of the fractional excretion of sodium (FE_{Na}), which represents the percentage of filtered sodium excreted in the urine (only valid in oliguric patients)

$$FE_{Na} = \frac{(\text{Urine sodium} \div \text{ urine creatinine}) \times 100\%}{(\text{Serum sodium} \div \text{ serum creatinine})}$$

5. Renal ultrasonography to rule out obstructive uropathy (hydroureter and hydronephrosis)
6. Complete blood count with differential and coagulation panel—to rule out systemic disease associated with ARF, including thrombotic thrombocytopenic purpura, hemolytic uremic syndrome, and disseminated intravascular coagulation
7. Urine eosinophils—eosinophiluria (urine eosinophils > 1%) may suggest AIN, although this test has poor sensitivity and specificity for this condition
8. Creatine phosphokinase—to rule out rhabdomyolysis
9. Serum calcium, phosphate, and magnesium—to rule out ARF-related electrolyte abnormalities

APPROACH TO ACUTE RENAL FAILURE

ARF is often multifactorial. The following guidelines provide a framework for determining the underlying cause(s) of ARF.

1. What Are the Laboratory Data?

a. Serum Creatinine

Using serum creatinine as an estimation of renal function has several important limitations:

(1) Small absolute increases in serum creatinine may represent large reductions in GFR.
(2) The serum creatinine concentration will not accurately reflect GFR in the

nonsteady state of ARF. Therefore, the Cockcroft-Gault equation, which estimates creatinine clearance based on age, ideal body weight, and serum creatinine should not be used in patients with ARF.

(3) Aggressive fluid hydration may dilute the serum creatinine, leading to an underestimation of the degree of renal failure.

(4) Creatinine is produced in muscle; therefore, levels may be normal or near-normal in ARF patients with low muscle mass or in the elderly.

(5) When GFR is low, there is increased tubular secretion of creatinine into the urine, underestimating the degree of renal failure.

(6) Some medications (such as trimethoprim and cimetidine) inhibit creatinine secretion into the urine without affecting GFR. For this reason, a rise in serum creatinine concentrations without a rise in blood urea nitrogen is not typically due to ARF.

b. The Blood Urea Nitrogen-to-Creatinine Ratio

Renal hypoperfusion causes increased tubular reabsorption of urea. As a result, the blood urea nitrogen-to-creatinine ratio should be > 20:1 in prerenal disease. However, this ratio is also elevated in conditions associated with an increased catabolic rate, including sepsis, gastrointestinal bleeding, and glucocorticoid use, even when renal hypoperfusion is absent.

c. Urine Sodium and Fractional Excretion of Sodium

The spot urine sodium concentration is usually below 20 mEq/L in patients with prerenal ARF but may be higher in the setting of diuretic use, osmotic diuresis, bicarbonaturia, and chronic renal disease (even if there is coexisting hypovolemia). In contrast, the spot urine sodium concentration is usually above 30 to 40 mEq/L in patients with ATN.

FE_{Na} should only be used in oliguric patients who do not have significant glycosuria and who have not recently received diuretics or mannitol.

In the appropriate setting, $FE_{Na} < 1\%$ suggests prerenal ARF with preservation of tubular reabsorption and renal concentrating ability whereas $FE_{Na} > 2\%$ suggests intrinsic renal disease (although most patients with contrast nephropathy have a low FE_{Na}).

2. Is the Renal Failure Acute or Chronic?

This determination is relatively easy when prior measurements of serum creatinine are available. Otherwise, findings suggestive of chronic renal failure include normocytic anemia, uremic bone disease, "half-and-half" nails (the lunula occupying approximately one half of the nail bed), and small kidneys (< 10 cm on renal ultrasound). However, small kidneys do not exclude an acute-on-chronic presentation of renal failure. In addition, some conditions (e.g., diabetes, amyloidosis, and obstruction) can cause an increase in kidney size.

3. What Are the Patient's Comorbidities?

Was there a recent vascular intervention or did the patient receive an intravenous contrast agent or other nephrotoxic medications? (See Table 17–1.)

a. Contrast Nephropathy

Contrast nephropathy is usually non-oliguric and typically presents with a rise in serum creatinine 24 to 48 hours after the contrast study. Creatinine generally peaks at 3 to 5 days and returns to baseline by 7 to 10 days.

b. Aminoglycosides

Aminoglycoside-induced ARF usually occurs after 1 week of therapy but can occur as soon as 1 to 2 days following initiation of therapy in patients with another renal insult. Single daily dosing of aminoglycosides appears to reduce the risk of nephrotoxicity compared to multiple daily dosing.

c. Atheroembolic Disease

Atheroembolic disease resulting from an invasive vascular procedure may cause symptoms immediately or symptoms can take months to appear. The diagnosis is confirmed when renal biopsy demonstrates cholesterol crystals in the renal vessels.

d. Allergic Interstitial Nephritis

The most common cause of AIN is a drug hypersensitivity reaction (see Table 17–1). AIN has a broad spectrum of presentation and can even occur in patients who have been tolerating the culprit medication for months or years. The classic triad of fever, rash, and eosinophilia is helpful when present but develops in less than one third of AIN patients. No single laboratory test can diagnose AIN; the gold standard is renal biopsy, which demonstrates an inflammatory cell infiltrate within the interstitium. Eosinophiluria, detected by Wright's stain or Hansel's stain, may suggest AIN but is nonspecific (eosinophiluria sometimes occurs in prostatitis, rapidly progressive glomerulonephritis, bladder carcinoma, and renal atheroembolic disease).

e. Hepatorenal Syndrome

Hepatorenal syndrome occurs predominantly in patients with liver failure and is characterized by severe reduction in renal blood flow and renal vasoconstriction. Hepatorenal syndrome is an unlikely diagnosis in patients without hyponatremia and ascites. Most patients also have a very low urine sodium concentration (< 10 mEq/L), but this finding cannot be used to reliably differentiate this syndrome from ATN. There are no conclusive diagnostic tests for hepatorenal syndrome. A fluid challenge (1500 mL isotonic saline) is recommended to rule out subtle volume depletion or overdiuresis.

Table 17-1. Drugs Associated with Acute Renal Failure

Mechanism	Examples
Alteration of intrarenal hemodynamics	NSAIDs, angiotensin-converting enzyme inhibitors, cyclosporine, tacrolimus, radiocontrast agents, amphotericin B
Direct tubular toxicity	Aminoglycosides, radiocontrast agents, cisplatin, cyclosporine, tacrolimus, amphotericin B, methotrexate, foscarnet, pentamidine, organic solvents, heavy metals
Heme-pigment-induced tubular toxicity (rhabdomyolysis)	Cocaine, ethanol, statins
Intratubular obstruction by precipitation of the drug, metabolites, or by-products	Acyclovir, sulfonamides, ethylene glycol, chemotherapy causing tumor lysis, methotrexate
Allergic interstitial nephritis	Penicillins, cephalosporins, sulfonamides, rifampin, ciprofloxacin, NSAIDs, thiazides, furosemide, cimetidine, phenytoin, allopurinol
Hemolytic–uremic syndrome	Cyclosporine, tacrolimus, cocaine, quinine

From Thadhani R, Pascual M, Bonventre JV. Acute renal failure. *N Engl J Med*. 1996;334:1448–1460. Copyright © 1996 Massachusetts Medical Society. All rights reserved. Adapted with permission, 2005. NSAIDs, nonsteroidal anti-inflammatory drugs.

4. What Is the Patient's Volume Status?

Adequate assessment of fluid status is usually obtained from the patient's medical history, physical examination, and hospital records for inpatients (daily weights, I/Os). Is there a history of nausea, vomiting, diarrhea, hemorrhage, overdiuresis, third-spacing of fluids (pancreatitis), heart failure, nephrotic syndrome, or cirrhosis? Are there postural signs, tachycardia, hypotension, and dry mucus membranes or are there crackles, elevated jugular venous pressure, ascites, and peripheral edema? For inpatients, what changes have occurred to the daily weights and fluid balance over the past few days? How much fluid was administered intraoperatively or postoperatively?

5. Are There Any Clues from the Urinalysis?

A urine specific gravity of 1.010 may be normal or may reflect loss of renal tubular concentrating and diluting capabilities. A bland urine sediment suggests renal hypoperfusion or obstructive uropathy. Urinalysis is usually also bland in patients with contrast nephropathy, although granular casts, tubular epithelial cells, and minimal proteinuria can be seen in this condition. The presence of brownish granular casts and tubular epithelial cells (muddy brown casts) suggests ATN. White cell casts can be seen in AIN and pyelonephritis. Red blood cell casts, dysmorphic red blood cells, and proteinuria suggest glomerulonephritis. Hematuria without red blood cells suggests rhabdomyolysis or hemolysis. Oxalate crystals occur in patients with ethylene glycol intoxication.

6. Does the Patient Have Urinary Obstruction?

A postrenal cause of ARF should be suspected in patients with prostatic disease, a solitary kidney, or intraabdominal (especially pelvic) tumors. Urine output cannot be used to exclude postrenal disease because these patients have a wide spectrum of presentation ranging from anuria to polyuria. Bladder catheterization will exclude bladder outlet obstruction (for example, from benign prostatic hypertrophy) but, unlike renal ultrasonography, will not rule out an obstruction at a site above the bladder. Renal ultrasonography should be performed early during the evaluation of ARF unless another obvious cause for ARF is found. Even in the setting of advanced cancer, ureteral stenting or percutaneous nephrostomy can relieve obstruction and improve short-term outcomes. A non-dilated collecting system does not fully exclude obstruction, especially if the obstruction is acute or there is coexisting hypovolemia or retroperitoneal fibrosis. Contrast studies of the urinary tract may be required in these settings if there is a high suspicion for obstruction.

TREATMENT

The following general management strategies are appropriate for all patients with ARF, regardless of cause:

1. Patients should start a "renal diet," which contains low amounts of sodium (2 g/day), phosphate, and potassium.
2. Adjust dosages of all medications metabolized or excreted by the kidneys. Formulas to estimate GFR are only accurate when renal function is stable. In ARF, all medications should be dosed for GFR < 10 mL/min.
3. If possible, discontinue nephrotoxins or substitute non-nephrotoxic alternatives. Monitor plasma levels of nephrotoxic drugs, such as cyclosporine and aminoglycosides.
4. Monitor fluid intake and output and measure body weight daily. Limit fluid intake in oliguric patients unless there is evidence of volume depletion.

5. Restore blood volume and blood pressure. Do not overzealously reduce blood pressures in patients with mild hypertension.

6. Monitor and aggressively treat infections (sepsis is the leading cause of death from ARF).

7. Monitor and treat complications of ARF, such as hyperkalemia, hyponatremia, and hyperphosphatemia. Hyperphosphatemia can be treated with calcium carbonate, calcium acetate, or phosphate binders (such as sevelamer). The calcium compounds should be given with meals; they bind dietary phosphate to form insoluble calcium phosphate, which is excreted in the stool. A potential side effect of the calcium-based agents is hypercalcemia. Limit administration of magnesium and magnesium-containing antacids to reduce the risk of hypermagnesemia.

ASPECTS OF TREATMENT UNIQUE TO THE UNDERLYING CAUSE OF RENAL FAILURE

1. Pre-Renal ARF

Pre-renal ARF is rapidly reversible if the underlying cause is promptly corrected before ATN develops.

2. Intrinsic ARF

a. Contrast Nephropathy

Patients with diabetes mellitus are at increased risk for contrast nephropathy. Therefore, most authorities recommend withholding metformin on the day of, and for 48 hours following, intravenous contrast administration because of the risk of lactic acidosis if ARF subsequently develops. N-acetylcysteine 600 mg twice daily on the day before and the day of the contrast study may reduce the risk of contrast nephropathy when given in conjunction with fluid hydration (such as one half normal saline or normal saline at 1 mL/kg/hr beginning 6 to 12 hours before contrast administration and continuing for 6 to 12 hours following contrast). If possible, diagnostic tests that do not require nephrotoxic contrast agents (such as magnetic resonance imaging or ultrasound) should be used in high-risk patients. Serum creatinine levels should be measured prior to contrast administration and 48 and 72 hours following contrast in patients at risk for contrast nephropathy.

b. Acute Tubular Necrosis

Non-oliguric ATN usually has a better prognosis than oliguric ATN. However, there are no therapies of proven benefit for either condition. Therefore, supportive care, avoidance of nephrotoxic insults, and maintenance of adequate renal hemodynamics should be emphasized while monitoring for complications of ARF and the need for dialysis.

c. Allergic Interstitial Nephritis

The most important intervention in AIN is discontinuation of the offending drug. Usually, treatment is supportive, although glucocorticoids and other immunosuppressive agents are sometimes used. Renal biopsy is usually recommended prior to initiating these therapies so that the diagnosis can be confirmed and the extent of fibrosis assessed. AIN is usually reversible if diagnosed promptly, but renal function can take weeks to return to baseline. The offending agent should be listed as a drug allergy in the medical record and the patient should be directly informed about this drug intolerance.

d. Rhabdomyolysis and Hemolysis

Heme pigments cause lipid peroxidation and free radical injury to the kidneys. This damage is prevented by alkalinization of the urine (assessed by measurement of urinary pH after the addition of sodium bicarbonate to the intravenous fluids), which stabilizes the reactive species. Forced alkalinization of the urine is also protective in patients with tumor lysis and methotrexate-mediated renal injury.

3. Post-Renal ARF

Prompt treatment of renal obstruction can lead to complete recovery of renal function, although the extent of recovery depends on the underlying disease. Post-obstructive diuresis may occur following correction of bilateral urinary obstruction. This condition is characterized by profuse diuresis (typically, 4–20 L/day), leading to hypovolemia, hypokalemia, and hypomagnesemia. Therefore, careful monitoring of fluid balance and electrolytes is mandatory in this setting.

DIURETICS AND RENAL DOSE DOPAMINE

Diuretics do not reduce mortality or the need for dialysis in patients with ARF. However, it is reasonable to try diuretics (e.g., furosemide 200 mg IV) in an attempt to convert oliguric ARF to non-oliguric ARF. If successful, this may simplify the management of ARF by reducing the risk of volume overload. Low-dose intravenous dopamine (1–3 µg/kg/min) increases renal blood flow and promotes natriuresis in healthy individuals, but "renal-dose" dopamine does not reduce mortality or promote recovery of renal function in patients with ARF.

WHEN TO START DIALYSIS

There are no absolute rules for starting dialysis, but proposed criteria include any of the following that are refractory to medical therapy: severe hyperkalemia with electrocardiographic changes, severe pulmonary edema, acidosis causing cardiac compromise (pH < 7.0), dialyzable toxins, and uremic complications (such as pericarditis or encephalopathy). Depending on the clinical scenario, the nephrologist may choose intermittent dialysis or continuous renal replacement therapy. There are no evidence-based guidelines on the optimum use of dialysis in ARF. Most patients with ARF do not require long-term dialysis.

WHEN TO CONSULT A NEPHROLOGIST

Nephrology consultation is appropriate if there is nephritic or nephrotic syndrome, unexplained ARF, rapidly worsening renal function, or potential for dialysis. Ideally, the nephrologist should be involved early in the patient's care rather than waiting until dialysis is imminent.

REFERENCES

Review Articles

1. Lameire N, Van Biesen W, Vanholder R. Acute renal failure. *Lancet* 2005;365:417–430.
2. Singri N, Ahya SN, Levin ML. Acute renal failure. *JAMA* 2003;289:747–751.
3. Thadhani R, Pascual M, Bonventre JV. Acute renal failure. *N Engl J Med*. 1996;334:1448–1460.

Etiology

1. Schrier RW, Wang W. Acute renal failure and sepsis. *N Engl J Med*. 2004;351:159–169.
2. Modi KS, Rao VK. Atheroembolic renal disease. *J Am Soc Nephrol*. 2001;12:1781–1787.
3. Esson ML, Schrier RW. Diagnosis and treatment of acute tubular necrosis. *Ann Intern Med*. 2002;137:744–752.
4. Murphy SW, Barrett BJ, Parfrey PS. Contrast nephropathy. *J Am Soc Nephrol*. 2000;11:177–182.

5. Gines P, Guevara M, Arroyo V, Rodes J. Hepatorenal syndrome. *Lancet* 2003;362:1819–1827.
6. Vanholder R, Sever MS, Erek E, Lameire N. Rhabdomyolysis. *J Am Soc Nephrol.* 2000;11:1553–1561.
7. Michel DM, Kelly CJ. Acute interstitial nephritis. *J Am Soc Nephrol.* 1998;9:506–515.

Treatment

1. Forni LG, Hilton PJ. Continuous hemofiltration in the treatment of acute renal failure. *N Engl J Med.* 1997;336:1303–1309.
2. Friedrich JO, Adhikari N, Herridge MS, Beyene J. Meta-analysis: Low-dose dopamine increases urine output but does not prevent renal dysfunction or death. *Ann Intern Med.* 2005;142:510–524.

CHAPTER 18

Hyperkalemia

KEY POINTS

1. Hyperkalemia is typically defined as a serum potassium concentration exceeding 5.0 to 5.5 mEq/L.

2. Hemolysis is the most common cause of pseudohyperkalemia (artifactual hyperkalemia that requires no treatment).

3. Potassium supplements, which are sometimes used in patients receiving diuretics and are often administered in the hospital as "potassium sliding scales," are a common cause of hyperkalemia.

4. Medications that inhibit the sodium–potassium–ATPase pump (digitalis, cyclosporine, tacrolimus, beta-blockers) reduce extracellular-to-intracellular potassium shifts and may cause hyperkalemia.

5. Renal excretion is the primary route of potassium elimination, which may be compromised by intrinsic renal disease, urinary tract obstruction, or hypoaldosteronism (adrenal insufficiency, angiotensin-converting enzyme inhibitors, angiotensin receptor blockers, heparin, cyclosporine).

6. Obtain an electrocardiogram (ECG), especially if the serum potassium ≥ 6.0 mEq/L.

7. The earliest ECG finding of hyperkalemia is narrowing and peaking ("tenting") of the T waves. Progressive hyperkalemia causes PR interval prolongation, P wave flattening, and QRS widening.

8. Intravenous calcium (10% calcium gluconate solution, 10 ml IV over 10 minutes, repeat in 5–10 minutes if no effect is seen) will not lower serum potassium concentrations but will stabilize the myocardium and is mandatory if there are ECG abnormalities attributable to the hyperkalemia.

9. The recommended first-line agent for the short-term treatment of hyperkalemia is 10 units of regular insulin IV (with 50 mL of 50% dextrose), but this therapy is temporary and must be followed by definitive therapy.

10. Definitive therapy includes sodium polystyrene sulfonate (15–30 gm orally 1–4 times/day), which eliminates potassium from the body but has a slow onset of action (at least 4 hours for full effect).

DEFINITION AND EPIDEMIOLOGY

Hyperkalemia is typically defined as a serum potassium concentration exceeding 5.0 to 5.5 mEq/L. Hyperkalemia occurs in up to 10% of hospitalized patients and can lead to life-threatening cardiac arrhythmias. Medications have been cited as a primary or contributing cause of up to 75% of inpatient hyperkalemia.

Etiology

Hyperkalemia occurs when

1. Potassium intake exceeds renal excretion, or
2. Potassium is shifted from the intracellular to extracellular compartment.

TRUE HYPERKALEMIA (Box 18-1)

Excessive Potassium Intake

Excessive potassium intake will rarely cause
hyperkalemia in healthy individuals with normal
renal function and no other contributing factors,
because the kidney can excrete hundreds of
milli-equivalents of potassium daily. However,
excessive potassium intake can exceed excretion
in patients with comorbidities predisposing to
hyperkalemia, such as renal failure. Therefore, as

Box 18-1. Nonmedication Causes of Hyperkalemia

> **Pseudohyperkalemia**
>
> Hemolysis
> Leukocytosis
> Thrombocytosis
> Prolonged tourniquet
> Potassium infusion near site of blood draw
> Laboratory error
>
> **Excessive Intake**
>
> Potassium supplement or dietary potassium
>
> **Extracellular Shift**
>
> Rhabdomyolysis
> Tissue necrosis (e.g., bowel infarction)
> Tumor lysis syndrome
> Metabolic acidosis
> Hyperosmolarity (mannitol, glucose)
> Intravascular hemolysis
> Hyperkalemic periodic paralysis
>
> **Reduced Renal Excretion**
>
> Renal insufficiency
> Urinary tract obstruction
> Hypoaldosteronism
> Reduced tubular excretion

a general rule of thumb, potassium sliding scales should not be used if the serum creatinine concentration is ≥ 2 mg/dL or if serum creatinine has increased by ≥ 0.5 mg/dL within 24 hours. Elderly patients with low muscle mass may have profound renal insufficiency with lower serum creatinine measurements. In these settings, and in patients receiving intravenous potassium (maximum infusion rate is 10 mEq/hr through a peripheral line and 20 mEq/hr through a central line), we do not administer more than 40 mEq potassium at any one time. In these patients, we obtain serum potassium measurements 2 hours after potassium supplementation to assess the adequacy of repletion and re-dose potassium, if necessary. Profound hypokalemia may require more aggressive treatment, including placement of a central venous catheter to administer potassium at a faster rate.

Intracellular to Extracellular Shift

Most potassium is located within cells, actively transported against a concentration gradient by the ubiquitous membrane-bound sodium–potassium–ATPase (Na–K–ATPase) pump. Therefore, medications that inhibit the Na–K–ATPase (digitalis, cyclosporine, tacrolimus, beta-blockers) will reduce potassium movement from the extracellular to intracellular compartment and may cause hyperkalemia (Table 18-1).

Reduced Renal Excretion

Renal excretion is the primary route of potassium removal from the body, and may be compromised by intrinsic renal disease, urinary tract obstruction, or hypoaldosteronism. Aldosterone, the final product of the renin–angiotensin system, promotes renal potassium secretion in the connecting segment and in the principal cells of the cortical collecting tubule. Therefore, adrenal insufficiency or drugs that reduce aldosterone production (angiotensin converting

Table 18-1. Common Drugs that Cause Hyperkalemia

Medication	Mechanisms
Angiotensin converting enzyme (ACE) inhibitors Angiotensin II receptor blocker (ARB) Nonsteroidal anti-inflammatory drugs	Reduces aldosterone production Decreases renal blood flow
Mineralocorticoid receptor antagonists (Spironolactone, eplerenone)	Reduces aldosterone action
Potassium-sparing diuretics (triamterene, amiloride) Trimethoprim (high-dose) Pentamidine	Reduces sodium reabsorption in the principal cell of the kidney
Potassium supplements Cyclosporine Tacrolimus (FK-506)	Excessive intake exceeding excretion Decreases aldosterone synthesis Reduces Na-K-ATPase activity
Heparin	Inhibits aldosterone production
Digitalis toxicity	Inhibits Na-K-ATPase
Beta-blockers	Inhibits renin secretion Reduces Na-K-ATPase activity Inhibits potassium channels in principle cells
Succinylcholine	Depolarizes cell membranes
Medicine salts (penicillin G)	High salt content
Insulin deficiency	Potassium redistribution from the intracellular space

Reprinted from Perazella MA, Drug-induced hyperkalemia: old culprits and new offenders, *Am J Med.* 109:307,2000, with permission from Excerpta Medica, Inc.

enzyme inhibitors, angiotensin receptor blockers, heparin, cyclosporine, tacrolimus) or antagonize the actions of aldosterone (spironolactone, eplerenone) may cause hyperkalemia. Other medications (nonsteroidal anti-inflammatory drugs) reduce potassium excretion by lowering renal blood flow and glomerular filtration rate. Some drugs (potassium-sparing diuretics, trimethoprim, pentamidine) cause hyperkalemia by inhibiting sodium reabsorption through the luminal membrane of the principal cell in the kidney, which reduces the electrical gradient for potassium secretion into the urine.

PSEUDOHYPERKALEMIA

Occasionally, a high potassium concentration is measured in the test tube when the true serum potassium level is normal. This condition is known as pseudohyperkalemia and requires no treatment. Hemolysis in the test tube after phlebotomy is the most common cause of this artifact, but is an unlikely explanation of apparent hyperkalemia if the serum does not have a visible color change. Pseudohyperkalemia can also occur when potassium is released inside the test tube from large numbers of leukocytes (usually $>70,000/cm^3$) or platelets (usually $>500,000/cm^3$), or when potassium is infused near the site of the blood draw. Pseudohyperkalemia is confirmed if the abnormal serum potassium concentration is more than 0.3 mEq/L higher than a simultaneously measured plasma potassium concentration (obtained using a "green-top" test tube or heparinized blood-gas syringe).

Initial Laboratory Testing

Initial laboratory testing should include:

1. Electrolytes (including repeat potassium), renal function (blood urea nitrogen and creatinine), and glucose

2. Electrocardiogram (ECG), especially if serum potassium $\geq$ 6.0 mEq/L
3. Digoxin level, if applicable
4. Arterial blood gas (if acidosis is suspected)
5. Complete blood count (if leukocytosis or thrombocytosis is suspected)

SIGNS AND SYMPTOMS

Hyperkalemia is often asymptomatic and detected incidentally when blood testing or an ECG is performed for other reasons. The earliest ECG finding of hyperkalemia is narrowing and peaking ("tenting") of the T waves, which may become tall (Fig. 18-1). With progressive hyperkalemia, the PR intervals become prolonged, the P waves become smaller and may disappear, and the QRS complexes widen (intraventricular conduction delay). Very severe hyperkalemia causes further widening of the QRS complexes, eventually leading to a large undulating (sine-wave) pattern and asystole.

The neuromuscular signs and symptoms of hyperkalemia are nonspecific and include generalized weakness, muscle cramps, paresthesias, delayed deep tendon reflexes, paralysis, and focal neurological deficits.

TREATMENT (Fig. 18-2)

Treatment of true hyperkalemia has four components (Table 18-2).

1. Protect the Myocardium—Intravenous Calcium

Intravenous calcium will not lower serum potassium concentrations but is mandatory if there are ECG abnormalities attributable to the hyperkalemia. This medication antagonizes the adverse effects of hyperkalemia on myocardial

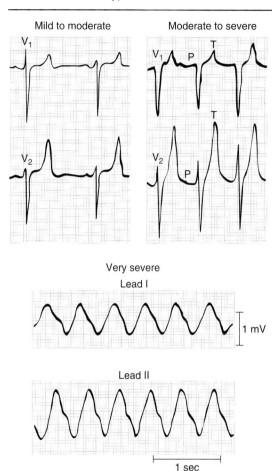

FIGURE 18-1. Electrocardiographic signs of hyperkalemia. The earliest change is peaking ("tenting") of the T waves. With progressive increases in the serum potassium concentration, the QRS complexes widen, and the P waves decrease in amplitude and may disappear. A sine-wave pattern occurs with very severe hyperkalemia and will lead to asystole unless emergency therapy is given. Reproduced with permission from Goldberger AL. *Clinical Electrocardiography: A Simplified Approach,* 6th ed. St. Louis: Mosby, 1999. p. 117.

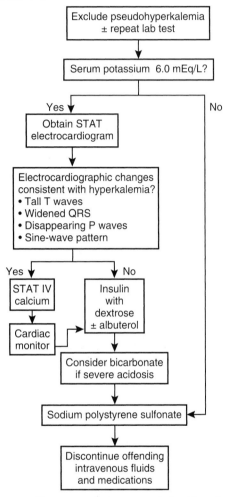

FIGURE 18–2. Recommended treatment algorithm for hyperkalemia.

repolarization and the conduction system, even in normocalcemic patients. Calcium gluconate is preferred, because calcium chloride must be given through a central line and can cause tissue necrosis if there is extravasation. The calcium dose should be repeated if there are no

Table 18-2. Treatment Options for Hyperkalemia

Drug	Dose	Mechanism	Onset of Action	Duration of Action	Potassium Reduction (mEq/L)
Calcium	10% calcium gluconate solution, 10 ml IV over 10 min (can repeat in 5–10 min if no effect is seen)	Antagonizes membrane depolarization	1–3 min	30–60 min	None
Insulin	Regular insulin, 10 U IV Add dextrose 50%, 50 ml IV if plasma glucose <250 mg/dl	Increases cellular potassium uptake	30 min	4–6 hr	0.5–1.2
Bicarbonate	1 ampule over 5 min Only recommended if severe, coexisting acidosis	Increases cellular potassium uptake	30 min	3 hr	?
Albuterol	Nebulized albuterol 10 mg	Increases cellular potassium uptake	30 min	2–6 hr	0.5–1.0
Sodium polystyrene sulfonate	15–30 gm orally one to four times daily in 20% sorbitol, or 30–50 gm per retention enema without sorbitol	Eliminates potassium	4–6 hr (1 hour if enema)	—	Varies

Continued

Table 18-2. Treatment Options for Hyperkalemia—cont'd

Drug	Dose	Mechanism	Onset of Action	Duration of Action	Potassium Reduction (mEq/L)
IV Loop Diuretic	Furosemide 20–200 mg IV (depending on renal function and whether the patient is diuretic naïve)	Eliminates potassium	At onset of diuresis	–	Varies
Hemodialysis	As tolerated	Eliminates potassium	Immediate	During dialysis	Varies

Adapted from Mount DB, Zandi-Nejad K. Disorders of potassium balance. In: Brenner BM, editor. *Brenner & Rector's The Kidney*, 7th ed. Philadelphia: WB Saunders; 2004. pp. 997–1040.

improvement in the ECG after 5 to 10 minutes. Because hypercalcemia may potentiate the myocardial toxicity of digitalis, intravenous calcium should be infused slowly (over 20–30 min) in hyperkalemic patients taking digitalis. Cardiac monitoring is indicated when there are ECG changes from hyperkalemia or there is a possibility that the hyperkalemia may worsen.

2. Shift Potassium from the Extracellular to Intracellular Domain

The recommended first-line agent for the short-term treatment of hyperkalemia is 10 units of regular insulin IV with 50 mL of 50% dextrose, which temporarily redistributes potassium from the extracellular to intracellular compartment (see Table 18-2). Dextrose should not be given to hyperglycemic patients (glucose concentrations ≥250 mg/dL).

Beta-2 agonists shift potassium intracellularly by activating the Na–K–ATPase, but are not effective in some patients with end-stage renal disease. Inhaled albuterol (10–20 mg nebulized in 4 mL of normal saline over 10 min) should not be used as monotherapy for hyperkalemia but can be combined with insulin and glucose for additive effects on serum potassium concentrations. Beta-2 agonists may cause tachycardia; therefore this class of medications should be used with caution in patients with coronary artery disease.

Bicarbonate has fallen out of favor for treatment of hyperkalemia because of questionable efficacy and the concern for volume overload in patients with renal failure. Bicarbonate may be reasonable in hyperkalemic patients with concurrent severe acidosis.

3. Increase Potassium Excretion

Potassium redistribution into the intracellular compartment is temporary and hyperkalemia will recur unless potassium is eliminated from the body. Although loop diuretics and thiazides may increase urinary potassium excretion, the resin sodium polystyrene sulfonate, which exchanges sodium for potassium in the gastrointestinal tract, is more commonly used. Sodium polystyrene sulfonate has a slow onset of action (at least 4 hours for full effect). Therefore, rapid potassium lowering with medications that cause potassium redistribution is often mandated while awaiting the full effects of the resin.

Sodium polystyrene sulfonate can be administered either orally or as a retention enema. The oral formulation is usually combined with 20% sorbitol to prevent constipation. Rectal administration of sorbitol is not recommended because several case reports have described subsequent colonic perforation, possibly due to mucosal dehydration from fluid loss into the colon lumen.

Dialysis is the most rapid method for treating hyperkalemia and is appropriate when renal function is markedly impaired and hyperkalemia is persistent and severe. However, initiating dialysis may take considerable time, especially if new venous access is required. Therefore, other treatments are appropriate while awaiting dialysis in an attempt to prevent further worsening of the hyperkalemia.

4. Determine the Etiology for the Hyperkalemia

Review medications and potassium intake (oral and intravenous). Assess renal function and search for non-medication causes of the hyperkalemia.

REFERENCES

Textbook Chapters

Mount DB, Zandi-Nejad K. Disorders of potassium balance. In: Brenner BM, editor.

Brenner & Rector's The Kidney, 7th ed.
Philadelphia: WB Saunders; 2004, pp. 997–1040.

Review Articles

Gennari FJ. Disorders of potassium homeostasis:
Hypokalemia and hyperkalemia. *Crit Care
Clin*. 2002;18:273–288.

Pathogenesis

Perazella MA. Drug-induced hyperkalemia:
Old culprits and new offenders. *Am J Med*.
2000;109:307–314.

Treatment

Kamel KS, Wei C. Controversial issues in the
treatment of hyperkalaemia. *Nephrol Dial
Transplant* 2003;18:2215–2218.

CHAPTER 19

Hyponatremia

KEY POINTS

1. Hyponatremia is defined as a serum sodium concentration below 135 mmol/L.
2. Hyponatremia is the most common electrolyte abnormality in hospitalized patients.
3. Patients with pseudohyponatremia have a normal serum sodium concentration, but the measured sodium level is falsely low. This artifact occurs when flame emission spectrometry is used to measure the serum sodium concentration in patients with severe hypertriglyceridemia or hyperparaproteinemia. Currently, most labs measure serum sodium with a sodium-selective electrode method, which does not cause this artifact.
4. Evaluation of hyponatremia involves assessment of volume status.
5. In hypovolemic hyponatremia the urine sodium concentration is usually <20 mmol/L, but may be higher in some settings, such as with diuretic use.
6. Euvolemic hyponatremia can occur in patients with hypothyroidism, adrenal insufficiency, a reset osmostat, and the syndrome of inappropriate secretion of antidiuretic hormone (SIADH).
7. Causes of SIADH include medications, tumors, and pulmonary or neurological disease. In SIADH, the urine is inappropriately concentrated and the spot urine sodium concentration is usually >30 mEq/L. A diagnosis of SIADH requires exclusion of thyroid, adrenal, and renal dysfunction.

8. Hypervolemic hyponatremia can occur in patients with heart failure, cirrhosis, and the nephrotic syndrome. The urine sodium concentration is usually <20 mmol/L.

9. Hyperglycemia causes dilutional hyponatremia. The serum sodium is lowered by 1.6 mmol/L for every 100 mg/dL increase in blood glucose over 100 mg/dL.

10. Most patients with mild hyponatremia are asymptomatic. Symptoms of rapid-onset and more severe hyponatremia include nausea, vomiting, lethargy, headache, restlessness, disorientation, and muscle cramps.

11. Initial laboratory testing for patients with hyponatremia should include electrolytes with glucose, serum osmolality, spot urinary sodium concentration, and assessment of thyroid and adrenal function (if applicable). Spot urine osmolality is only sometimes helpful because almost all cases of hyponatremia are associated with inappropriately concentrated urine.

12. Cerebral edema can occur when acute (<48 hours) hyponatremia is not treated promptly and may cause increased intracranial pressure, seizures, coma, tentorial herniation, and death.

13. There is no consensus about the optimal treatment of acute, symptomatic hyponatremia. One proposed management plan is to initially raise the serum sodium by 2 mmol/L per hour using hypertonic (3%) saline.

14. Depending on the clinical circumstances, treatment options for patients with chronic (>48 hours) hyponatremia include fluid restriction, intravenous saline, oral salt tablets, and medications, such as demeclocycline and loop diuretics.

15. Fluid restriction is usually the most appropriate treatment for SIADH in

addition to therapy directed at the underlying cause. Administration of normal saline can worsen the hyponatremia of SIADH.

16. With chronic hyponatremia, the sodium should be raised by, at most, 0.5 mmol/L/hr unless there are severe symptoms. In all cases of chronic hyponatremia, the sodium should be raised by no more than 12 mmol/L/day.

17. Neuronal demyelination (myelinolysis) is a devastating neurologic complication that can occur when chronic hyponatremia is corrected too quickly.

DEFINITIONS

Hyponatremia: Serum sodium concentration <135 mmol/L.

Osmolality: The concentration of solutes (measured in osmoles) per kilogram of water. Usually, sodium is the most important contributor to serum osmolality.

Effective osmolality (tonicity): Substances that contribute to osmolality but cannot move freely across cell membranes. These solutes (such as mannitol and sodium) cause water to move across membranes by osmosis until similar osmolalities are achieved on both sides of the membranes.

Ineffective osmolality: Substances that contribute to osmolality but easily cross cell membranes. These solutes (such as urea and ethanol) do not cause movement of water across membranes, because the solutes themselves can cross membranes until similar osmolalities are achieved on both sides of the membranes.

Hypotonic hyponatremia: Low serum tonicity/effective osmolality PLUS low serum sodium concentration. These patients may have normal or high serum osmolality if there are sufficient amounts of ineffective osmoles (e.g., concurrent ethanol intoxication). Patients with acute hypotonic hyponatremia are at risk for cerebral edema because the reduced effective osmolality of the serum will cause movement of water by osmosis into neurons.

EPIDEMIOLOGY

Hyponatremia is the most common electrolyte abnormality in hospitalized patients, and the syndrome of inappropriate secretion of anti-diuretic hormone (SIADH) is the most common cause of hyponatremia in this patient population.

Pseudohyponatremia

Patients with pseudohyponatremia have normal serum sodium concentrations, but the measured sodium level is falsely low. This artifact occurs when flame emission spectrometry is used to measure the serum sodium concentration in patients with severe hypertriglyceridemia or hyperparaproteinemia (e.g., multiple myeloma). Currently, most labs measure serum sodium with a sodium-selective electrode method, which does not cause this artifact. A normal osmolal gap excludes pseudohyponatremia (see "Approach to Finding the Cause of Hyponatremia" on p. 353).

PATHOPHYSIOLOGY

True hyponatremia occurs when there is either water retention or, less commonly, sodium loss. The pathophysiology of hyponatremia is easiest to conceptualize when patients are classified according to volume status.

Reduced Extracellular Volume

Hypovolemia of any cause (vomiting, diarrhea, diuretics, and excessive sweating) leads to sodium and water depletion. Appropriate compensatory activation of the renin–angiotensin–aldosterone system and antidiuretic hormone production leads to sodium and water reabsorption by the kidneys. Hyponatremia occurs when the sodium deficit exceeds the water deficit. Drinking hypotonic fluid, such as water or tea, can exacerbate the hyponatremia.

Normal or Near-Normal Extracellular Volume

Euvolemic hyponatremia can occur in patients with hypothyroidism, adrenal insufficiency, a reset osmostat, and SIADH.

Box 19-1. Causes of the Syndrome of Inappropriate Secretion of Antidiuretic Hormone

Cancer

Pulmonary tumors
Mediastinal tumors
Extrathoracic tumors

Central Nervous System Disorders

Acute psychosis
Mass lesions
Inflammatory and demyelinating diseases
Stroke
Hemorrhage
Trauma

Medications

Desmopressin
Nicotine
Phenothiazines
Tricyclic antidepressants
Selective serotonin reuptake inhibitors

Medications—

Opiate derivatives
Chlorpropamide
Clofibrate
Carbamazepine
Cyclophosphamide
Vincristine
Nonsteroidal anti-inflammatory drugs (NSAIDs)

Pulmonary Conditions

Infections
Acute respiratory failure
Positive-pressure ventilation

Miscellaneous

Postoperative state
Pain
Severe nausea
Human immunodeficiency virus/AIDS

SIADH has many causes, including medications, pain, excessive nausea and vomiting, tumors, and pulmonary or neurological disease (Box 19-1). These conditions either stimulate antidiuretic hormone release or increase the kidneys' response to antidiuretic hormone. As a result, there is inappropriate retention of free water, dilution of normal extracellular amounts of sodium, and subsequent development of hyponatremia. SIADH does not typically cause clinically apparent volume overload because most of the retained free water moves into the intracellular compartment and does not remain in the bloodstream and interstitium.

The reset osmostat syndrome, a rare cause of hyponatremia, occurs when there is a lowering of

the osmolality threshold that stimulates antidiuretic hormone release. These patients often
have long-standing, disabling conditions, such as
tuberculosis, quadriplegia, and psychosis, and
tend to have chronically low but stable serum
sodium concentrations. These patients can normally excrete a water load and achieve normal
maximal urine dilution (these criteria are used to
diagnose the syndrome). These patients are also
able to concentrate the urine at serum
osmolalities above the reset level.

Psychogenic polydipsia is an unusual cause of
hyponatremia that is typically seen in patients with
schizophrenia or other psychiatric diseases.
Hyponatremia in this setting results from large
ingestion of free water over a short time period.
When renal function is normal, ingestion of more
than 20 L/day is needed to cause hyponatremia by
overcoming the kidneys' ability to excrete the water.

Expanded Extracellular Volume

Hypervolemic hyponatremia is usually caused
by heart failure, cirrhosis, and the nephrotic
syndrome. Although these patients are volume
overloaded, they typically have reduced effective
circulating blood volume and poor renal perfusion. As a result, there is release of antidiuretic
hormone from the posterior pituitary (which
causes water retention by the kidneys) and activation of the renin–angiotensin–aldosterone
system (which causes the kidneys to avidly retain
sodium). Therefore, these patients have an
increased amount of body sodium and water.
Hyponatremia occurs if the increase in sodium is
less than the increase in water.

SYMPTOMS AND SIGNS

Most patients with mild hyponatremia (serum
sodium concentration >125 mmol/L) are
asymptomatic. Lower serum sodium concentrations are more likely to cause symptoms, espe-

cially if the onset of hyponatremia is rapid. Typical symptoms include nausea, vomiting, lethargy, headache, restlessness, disorientation, and muscle cramps. On physical exam, reflexes may be diminished. Patients with acute, severe hypotonic hyponatremia are at risk for cerebral edema, which can cause increased intracerebral pressure, seizures, coma, tentorial herniation, respiratory depression, and death. Therefore, rapid correction of the serum sodium concentration is appropriate if there are neurological findings consistent with hyponatremia (see "Treatment").

Laboratory Data

Initial laboratory testing for patients with hyponatremia should include the following (obtaining some of these tests may depend on clinical circumstances):

1. **Electrolytes** (with repeat sodium measurement to rule out lab error) and **glucose** (to rule out hyperglycemia)
2. **Serum osmolality**—A low value confirms true hypo-osmolality; a normal or high osmolality does not necessarily exclude hypotonicity
3. **Spot urinary sodium concentration**
4. **Spot urine osmolality** is only sometimes helpful because almost all cases of hyponatremia are associated with inappropriately concentrated urine. Maximally dilute urine (urine osmolality <100 mOsm/kg H_2O) in the setting of hyponatremia implies appropriate and complete suppression of antidiuretic hormone and occurs in psychogenic polydipsia and the reset osmostat syndrome.
5. **Serum uric acid and blood urea nitrogen (BUN)**—Low values are suggestive of euvolemia and SIADH rather than hypovolemia.

6. When there is clinical suspicion for thyroid or adrenal dysfunction or to establish a diagnosis of SIADH

   (a) **Serum thyrotropin (TSH)**—Serum thyroxine levels should also be measured if a pituitary or hypothalamic cause of hypothyroidism is suspected because serum TSH may be normal or only modestly elevated in those settings.

   (b) **Cortrosyn stimulation test** (see Chapter 4)

APPROACH TO FINDING THE CAUSE OF HYPONATREMIA (Fig. 19-1)

Is There Laboratory Error?

The sodium measurement should be presumed accurate in patients with signs and symptoms consistent with hyponatremia. However, a very low sodium concentration in a patient who is otherwise clinically well may be a laboratory error. In this case, ensure that the blood collection was not obtained from a vein that was simultaneously receiving an infusion of hypotonic solution and repeat the measurement.

Rule Out Hyperglycemia and Assess Plasma Osmolality

Elevated blood glucose causes an osmotic shift of water from the intracellular to the extracellular compartment. Therefore, hyperglycemia can cause dilution of serum sodium concentrations and hyponatremia. The serum sodium declines by approximately 1.6 mmol/L for every 100 mg/dL increase in blood glucose concentrations over 100 mg/dL. The corrected sodium (Na) can be calculated as follows:

$$\text{Na (corrected)} = \text{Measured Na} + \frac{1.6 \times (\text{glucose [mg/dL]} - 100 \, \text{mg/dL})}{100}$$

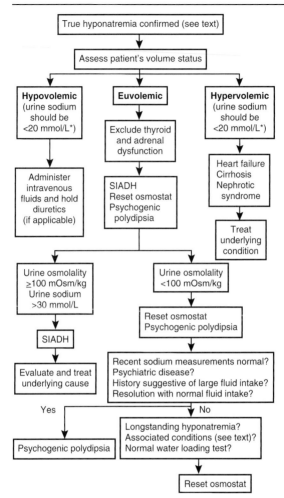

FIGURE 19–1. Approach to the patient with hyponatremia. *Spot urine sodium may be higher in the setting of diuretic use, osmotic diuresis, bicarbonaturia, and chronic kidney disease even if there is coexisting hypovolemia or reduced effective circulating blood volume.

SIADH, syndrome of inappropriate secretion of antidiuretic hormone.

The reduced contribution of sodium to the serum osmolality is offset by the contribution of the elevated glucose. This is evident from the formula used to calculate plasma osmolality (reference range 280–295 mOsm/kg H_2O):

$$Plasma\ osmolality(mOsm/kg\ H_2O =$$
$$(2 \times serum\ sodium\ [mmol/L]) +$$
$$(glucose\ [mg/dL] \div 18) + (BUN\ [mg/dL] \div 2.8)$$

These patients are usually not at risk for cerebral edema because serum tonicity is not typically reduced (glucose is an effective osmole in the setting of insulin deficiency).

The Osmolal Gap

When plasma osmolality is measured, the preceding formula can be used to calculate the "osmolal gap" as follows:

$$Osmolal\ gap = Measured\ plasma\ osmolality -$$
$$Calculated\ plasma\ osmolality$$

An osmolal gap >10 mOsm/kg H_2O implies the presence of osmotically active substances in the bloodstream other than sodium, glucose, and urea. Possibilities include:

(1) Pseudohyponatremia
(2) The presence of another effective osmole, such as mannitol, glycine, or sorbitol
(3) The presence of another ineffective osmole, such as ethanol, methanol, or ethylene glycol

Determine the Patient's Fluid Status

Adequate assessment of fluid status can usually be obtained by a combination of the patient history, physical examination, and hospital records for inpatients (daily weights, I/Os). Volume status provides a framework for determining the cause of the patient's hyponatremia (Table 19-1).

Table 19-1. Causes of Hyponatremia According to Volume Status

Hypovolemic		Euvolemic	Hypervolemic
Renal sodium loss	**Extra-renal sodium loss**		
Diuretics (esp. thiazides)	Diarrhea	Hypothyroidism	Heart failure
Osmotic diuresis	Vomiting	Adrenal insufficiency	Cirrhosis
Mineralocorticoid deficiency	Blood loss	SIADH	Nephrotic syndrome
Salt-wasting nephropathy	Excessive sweating	Reset osmostat syndrome	Renal failure
Bicarbonaturia	Third-spacing of fluids (pancreatitis, burns, trauma)	Decreased intake of solutes	Pregnancy
Ketonuria		Beer potomania	
		Tea-and-toast diet	

SIADH, syndrome of inappropriate secretion of antidiuretic hormone.
From Adrogue HJ, Madias NE, Hyponatremia. *N Engl J Med.* 2000;342:1581-1589. Copyright © 2000 Massachusetts Medical Society. All rights reserved. Adapted with permission, 2005.

Reduced Extracellular Volume

Does the patient have a history of vomiting, diarrhea, diuretic use (the timeframe for thiazide-induced hyponatremia is usually within 14 days of starting therapy), or excessive sweating? On physical examination, there may be postural signs, tachycardia, hypotension, dry mucus membranes, poor skin turgor (loss of normal skin elasticity manifested by slow sagging of the skin back into position after being pinched up into a fold), and low jugular venous pressure. Appropriate activation of the renin–angiotensin–aldosterone system causes avid sodium retention by the kidneys. As a result, the urine sodium concentration is typically below 20 mmol/L and the urine output should be reduced. The spot urine sodium concentration may be higher in the setting of diuretic use, osmotic diuresis, bicarbonaturia, and chronic renal disease even if there is coexisting hypovolemia.

Normal or Near-Normal Extracellular Volume

Does the patient have signs or symptoms of hypothyroidism or adrenal insufficiency (these disorders impair free water clearance)? Thyroid, adrenal, and renal dysfunction must be excluded before considering a diagnosis of SIADH or the reset osmostat syndrome. Patients with SIADH have an inappropriately concentrated urine (urine osmolality >100 mOsm/kg H_2O) and a urine sodium concentration >30 mEq/L (urine sodium may be lower in patients on a low-sodium diet).

The reset osmostat syndrome is formally diagnosed with a water load challenge. These patients will excrete the water normally and achieve maximal dilution of the urine (urine osmolality <100 mOsm/kg H_2O).

Psychogenic polydipsia can be differentiated from the preceding conditions by medical history and by measuring the urine osmolality. A random measurement will show an appropriately dilute urine osmolality (<100 mOsm/kg H_2O) consistent with suppression of endogenous antidiuretic hormone production.

Expanded Extracellular Volume

Does the patient have signs or symptoms of heart failure, cirrhosis, or the nephrotic syndrome? Heart failure is suggested by a history of orthopnea, dyspnea, and lower extremity edema with or without chest pain. Physical examination may reveal elevated jugular venous pressure, pulmonary crackles, and lower extremity edema. Cirrhosis may be present in patients with a history of any or all of the following: encephalopathy, ascites, jaundice, abnormal liver function tests, hypoalbuminemia, and elevated prothrombin time. Nephrotic syndrome is characterized by more than 3 gm of proteinuria per day. Loss of albumin and other oncotic proteins causes third-spacing of fluids and peripheral edema.

Because effective circulating blood volume is reduced in these conditions, the kidneys attempt to avidly retain sodium. As a result, spot urinary sodium concentrations are usually below 20 mmol/L (provided the patient is not concurrently receiving a diuretic).

Review Medications and Intravenous Fluid Orders

If applicable, assess how much free water has been recently administered through intravenous fluids and intravenous medications (for example, antibiotics mixed with water). Is the patient getting diuretics or other medications that cause hyponatremia (see Box 19-1 and Table 19-1)?

TREATMENT

General Principles

Acute, Symptomatic Hyponatremia

Patients with acute (<48 hr), symptomatic hyponatremia are at risk for cerebral edema and permanent brain injury if the hyponatremia is not treated promptly. The first steps should be to ensure that the airway is protected and to administer an anti-epileptic drug, if needed. There is no consensus about the optimal treatment of symptomatic hyponatremia. One proposed treatment plan is to raise the serum sodium by 2 mmol/L/hr using hypertonic (3%) saline until life-threatening symptoms resolve, there is improvement in symptoms, or the serum

---

Box 19-2. Calculating Infusion Rates for Intravenous Fluids When Treating Hyponatremia

Step 1: Choose an intravenous fluid (this will usually be normal saline or, in cases of severe hyponatremia, 3% normal saline).

Intravenous Fluid	Sodium Content (mmol/L)
Normal saline (NS)	154
1/2 NS	77
1/4 NS	39
3% NS	513
5% dextrose in NS (D5NS)	154
5% dextrose in 1/2 NS (D5 1/2 NS)	77
5% dextrose in water (D5W)	0
10% dextrose in water (D10W)	0

Step 2: Determine the patient's "total body water" content.

Total body water (L) =
    Fraction from following table × weight (kg)

Children	0.60
Women	
Non-elderly	0.50
Elderly	0.45
Men	
Non-elderly	0.60
Elderly	0.50

Step 3: Estimate the effect of 1 L of your chosen intravenous fluid on the serum sodium concentration.

Serum sodium change=

$$\frac{(\text{sodium content} + \text{potassium content}) - \text{serum sodium}}{\text{Total body water (from Step 2)} + 1}$$

Step 4: Determine the rate of sodium correction (in mmol/L/hr) you desire based on the presence of symptoms and the chronicity of the hyponatremia.

Step 5: Divide the rate from Step 4 by the result from Step 3, then multiply by 1000. This is the desired rate of infusion per hour (in mL) of your selected intravenous fluid.

An example: Suppose your patient developed a serum sodium concentration of 114 mmol/L 1 day following general surgery and is having seizures. You decide to treat with hypertonic saline, which has a sodium concentration of 513 mmol/L (Step 1). You patient is a middle-aged man who weights 70 kg, so his total body water is $0.6 \times 70 = 42$ L (Step 2). The effect of 1 L of hypertonic saline will be to increase the serum sodium concentration by ($[513 + 0] - 114$) $\div$ ($42 + 1$) $= 9.28$ mmol/L (Step 3). You decide to initially correct the serum sodium concentration by 1 mmol/L/hr (Step 4). Therefore, the desired rate of infusion of hypertonic saline will be $1 \div 9.28 = 0.108$ L/hr, or 108 mL/hr (Step 5).

sodium concentration is increased above 125 mmol/L. Box 19-2 demonstrates how to calculate the rate of infusate needed to raise serum sodium concentrations by a desired amount. Co-administration of a loop diuretic, such as furosemide, will limit saline-induced volume expansion, enhance free water excretion, and accelerate the sodium correction. Sodium levels should be monitored every 1 to 2 hours to ensure appropriate correction.

Chronic Hyponatremia

Patients with chronic (>48 hr) hyponatremia are at risk for myelinolysis if the sodium is corrected too rapidly. Depending on the cause and clinical circumstances, treatment options include fluid restriction, administration of intravenous saline (see Box 19-2), oral salt tablets, and medications, such as demeclocycline and loop diuretics (not thiazides). Whichever method is used, the serum sodium should not be increased by more than 0.5 mmol/L per hour. One exception is if the patient has severe symptoms, such as seizures, obtundation, or coma. The sodium concentration in these patients should be increased by 4 to 6 mmol/L over the first 1 to 2 hours; then, the rate of increase should be slowed to 0.5 to 1 mmol/L/hr. The infusion should be stopped when the patient becomes asymptomatic, regardless of the degree of hyponatremia. In all cases of chronic hyponatremia, the serum sodium should not be increased by more than 12 mmol/L/day.

Other Treatment Considerations

Potassium

Hypokalemia leads to potassium movement from the intracellular to extracellular spaces. To maintain electroneutrality, sodium moves intracellularly. Correction of hypokalemia will move some of the intracellular sodium back into the extracellular space as potassium reenters the cells. Therefore, a greater-than-anticipated increase in the serum sodium concentration will occur when patients with concurrent hyponatremia and hypokalemia are given normal saline with added potassium, as opposed to normal saline only.

Reduced Extracellular Volume

Diuretics should be temporarily discontinued or the long-term dose should be reduced (if applicable) and the patient should receive intravenous fluid. When the hyponatremia is mild, supportive care is usually all that is needed for self-limited conditions, such as vomiting and diarrhea from gastroenteritis.

Normal or Near-Normal Extracellular Volume

Hyponatremia due to thyroid or adrenal dysfunction should improve with the appropriate hormone therapy. Fluid restriction (sometimes to less than 1 L/day) is the most appropriate treatment for SIADH in addition to therapy directed at the underlying cause. Administration of normal saline can worsen the hyponatremia of SIADH because the infused salt can be excreted in concentrated urine, leading to a net retention of water. A small fluid challenge, such as 500 mL normal saline, can be administered intravenously in carefully selected patients when other available data fail to differentiate SIADH from mild hypovolemia. SIADH is more likely if the serum sodium worsens or remains unchanged with this intervention whereas hypovolemia is more likely if the serum sodium improves.

In specific settings, demeclocycline (600–1200 mg/day) can be used to control hyponatremia. Demeclocycline induces nephrogenic diabetes insipidus by inhibiting the action of antidiuretic hormone on the kidneys. When diuresis begins, the patient must have free access to water; otherwise, hypernatremia will occur. After the initial response, the dose should be reduced to the lowest amount needed to normalize the serum sodium during unrestricted access to fluid. Potential side effects include nephrotoxicity (especially in patients with liver disease) and photosensitivity. Given these complex issues, we recommend consultation with a subspecialist when considering demeclocycline therapy.

Expanded Extracellular Volume

Treatment directed at the underlying condition (e.g., angiotensin-converting enzyme inhibitors and loop diuretics for heart failure) should improve the sodium concentration.

COMPLICATIONS

The most important complications of hyponatremia are acute cerebral edema and myelinolysis. Patients at risk for cerebral edema include postoperative menstruating women and elderly women using thiazide diuretics. Groups at risk for myelinolysis include burn patients, alcoholics, malnourished individuals, and elderly women using thiazide diuretics. Both complications are related to the brain's underlying adaptive response to hyponatremia.

The Brain and Hyponatremia

A reduction in the effective osmolality of the extracellular space causes movement of water into cells and increases intracellular volumes. The brain's earliest defense against cerebral edema involves shunting of some of the extracellular fluid into the systemic circulation via the cerebrospinal fluid. Thereafter, the brain attempts to reduce intracellular osmolality by losing intracellular potassium and then organic osmolytes, such as myoinositol phosphocreatine and amino acids.

Cerebral Edema

Cerebral edema can occur when acute hyponatremia is untreated or treated too slowly. If the preceding adaptive mechanisms fail, the brain may expand against the rigid cranium, leading to increased intracranial pressure and cerebral herniation.

Patients at risk for cerebral edema have low *effective* plasma osmolality, but the overall plasma osmolality (effective + ineffective osmoles) may be normal. The presence of ineffective osmoles (e.g., urea from renal failure) does not alter the risk of cerebral edema, because these osmoles do not cause water movement across membranes (the osmoles themselves easily move across cell membranes).

Myelinolysis

The process of brain adaptation to hyponatremia also accounts for the risk of myelinolysis when chronic hyponatremia is corrected too quickly. In this setting, a rapid increase in extracellular osmolality causes movement of intracellular fluid from the adapted brain cells to the extracellular space. As a result, the brain cells shrink and demyelination of the pontine and extrapontine neurons may occur. This rare complication can develop one to several days after aggressive treatment of hyponatremia and has a broad range of neurological symptoms, including seizures, ataxia, dystonia, coma, quadriplegia, pseudobulbar palsy (injury to the upper motor neurons of the corticobulbar tracts that causes dysarthria, dysphagia, dysphonia, impaired tongue and facial movement, and emotional lability), and death. Myelinolysis is usually a clinical diagnosis although there are some characteristic MRI findings (symmetric pontine and extra-pontine lesions that are hyperintense on T2-weighted images and hypointense on T1-weighted images). Other tests, such as brainstem auditory evoked potentials, can be useful. Most patients have persistent neurological deficits. Myelinolysis rarely occurs in patients with a serum sodium above 120 mmol/L or in patients with acute hyponatremia.

REFERENCES

Review Articles

1. Adrogue HJ, Madias NE. Hyponatremia. *N Engl J Med*. 2000;342:1581–1589.
2. Oster JR, Singer I. Hyponatremia, hyposmolality, and hypotonicity. Tables and fables. *Arch Intern Med*. 1999;159:333–336.
3. Yeates KE, Singer M, Morton AR. Salt and water: A simple approach to hyponatremia. *CMAJ* 2004;170:365–369.
4. Freda BJ, Davidson MB, Hall PM. Evaluation of hyponatremia: A little physiology goes a long way. *Cleve Clin J Med*. 2004;71:639–650.
5. Smith DM, McKenna K, Thompson CJ. Hyponatremia. *Clin Endocrinol*. 2000;52:667–678.
6. Kumar S, Berl T. Sodium. *Lancet* 1998;352:220–228.

Treatment

1. Lauriat S, Berl T. The hyponatremic patient: Practical focus on therapy. *J Am Soc Nephrol*. 1997;8:1599–1607.
2. Gross P, Reimann D, Henschkowski J, Damian M. Treatment of severe hyponatremia: Conventional and novel aspects. *J Am Soc Nephrol*. 2001;12:S10–S14.

Complications

Laureno R, Karp BI. Myelinolysis after correction of hyponatremia. *Ann Intern Med*. 1997;126:57–62.

Index

V